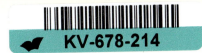

Selected papers of the VIIth International Congress of Radiology in
Oto-Rhino-Laryngology, Copenhagen, May 31 – June 2, 1976

Modern Methods of Radiology in ORL

Volume Editors
S. Brünner, Copenhagen and P. E. Andersen, Odense

145 figures, 15 tables, 1978

S. Karger · Basel · München · Paris · London · New York · Sydney

Advances in Oto-Rhino-Laryngology

Vol. 20: Otophysiology. International Symposium on Otophysiology. Eds.: J. E. Hawkins, jr.; M. Lawrence, and W. P. Work, Ann Arbor, Mich.
VI + 542 p., 289 fig., 18 tab., 1973. ISBN 3-8055-1338-0

Vol. 21: Radiology in Oto-Rhino-Laryngology. Ed.: S. Brünner, Copenhagen.
VIII + 156 p., 69 fig., 23 tab., 1974. ISBN 3-8055-1632-0

Vol. 22: Audio-Vestibular System and Facial Nerve. Ed.: W. J. Oosterveld, Amsterdam.
X + 220 p., 119 fig., 19 tab., 1977. ISBN 3-8055-2354-8

Vol. 23: Pediatric Otorhinolaryngology. Ed.: B. Jazbi, Kansas City, Mo.
VIII + 206 p., 101 fig., 16 tab., 1 cpl., 1978. ISBN 3-8055-2674-1

Cataloging in Publication
    International Congress of Radiology in ORL, Copenhagen 1976.
    Modern methods of radiology in ORL / volume editor, S. Brünner. – Basel, New York: Karger 1978.
    (Advances in oto-rhino-laryngology; v. 24)
    1. Otorhinolaryngologic Diseases – radiography 2. Tomography, Computerized Axial
    I. Brünner, Sam, ed. II. Title III. Series.
    W1 AD701 v. 24 / WV 150 I61m 1976
    ISBN 3-8055-2707-1

Modern Methods of Radiology in ORL

Advances in
Oto-Rhino-Laryngology

Vol. 24

Series Editor
C. R. Pfaltz, Basel

S. Karger · Basel · München · Paris · London · New York · Sydney

Contents

Contents

Editorial Introduction

The VIIth International Congress of Radiology in ORL took place in Copenhagen, in June 1976. The objective of this congress was to bring together some of the people who are well-known by their previous scientific papers and who show a special interest in radiology in ORL.

For the first time the computed axial tomography scanners have been discussed with a possibility to make progress in ORL diagnosis with less strain on the patient. A great number of papers are related to this subject. Well-known ORL specialized X-ray doctors have given their informations about the experiences in this field of X-ray diagnosis.

Undoubtedly this is a new area in radiology in ORL and the experiences to be achieved from these first papers concerning CAT scanners will increase and renew the research within this field in diagnostic radiology. The diagnostic possibilities with the polytome and the stratomatic machine in tomography of tumors of the rhinopharynx, lesion of the facial canal and in Menière's disease are discussed. It has been demonstrated that these apparatuses will improve and increase the diagnosis in our daily work.

Spring 1977   S. Brünner

Adv. Oto-Rhino-Laryng., vol. 24, pp. 1–8 (Karger, Basel 1978)

Computed Axial Tomography in Otorhinolaryngology

Enrique Palacios and Galdino Valvassori

Department of Radiology, Neuroradiology Section,
Loyola University of Chicago, Chicago, Ill., and Eye and Ear Infirmary,
Department of Radiology, University of Illinois, Urbana, Ill.

Computed tomography, the new noninvasive diagnostic procedure, considered to be a major breakthrough in modern diagnostic radiology, has definite indications in clinical problems in otorhinolaryngology (ORL).

The principles of computed tomography (CT) have been discussed at length in the literature [1–3, 6, 9, 10]. The purpose of this communication is to illustrate briefly the usefulness and applications of CT in ORL. Our experience consists of over 9,000 examinations, carried out mainly with the first generation head unit.

Conventional methods, particularly multidirectional tomography, applied to ORL remain indispensable for the demonstration of bone detail. CT, however, allows improved evaluation of the soft tissues and their relationship to bony structures (fig. 1, 2).

The cerebellopontine angle (CPA) is an area where CT has proved to be of significant value, particularly in the diagnosis of acoustic neurinomas and meningiomas [5, 11]. Other lesions involving the CPA which have been detected by this method are listed on table I.

Acoustic neurinomas are demonstrated as dense masses. Obliteration or displacement of the fourth ventricle to the contralateral side due to mass effect may be seen with moderate and large size tumors (fig. 3). According to our experience and related data from other institutions, 95% of acoustic neurinomas, 2 cm in diameter or greater, are only visualized on CT by enhancement with intravenous injection of iodinated contrast medium (fig. 4). Tumors as small as 6–8 mm have been suspected on CT and subsequently proven to be present. At the present time, however, with the available units, tumors projecting less than 1.5–2.0 cm into the CPA may not be visualized by CT. Posterior fossa cisternogram in these cases must be done particularly

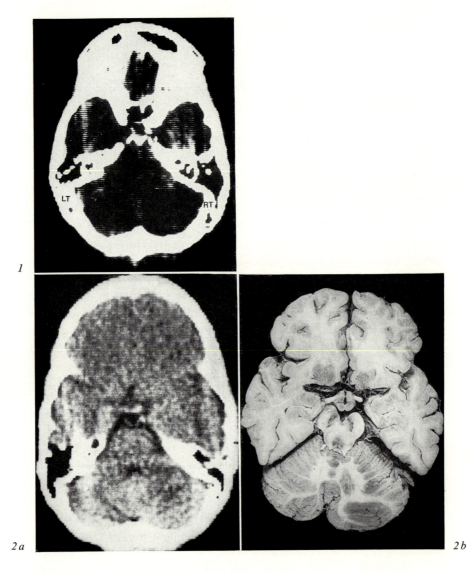

Fig. 1. CT demonstrated normal structures at the base of the skull. Note the mastoids and petrous portions of the temporal bones.

Fig. 2. a Computed tomogram at the level of the CPA demonstrating normal structures of the posterior fossa. b Normal brain section at similar level.

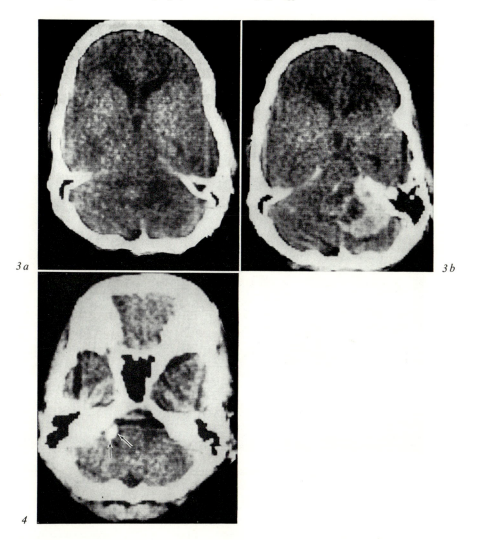

Fig. 3. Large acoustic neurinoma on the right. *a* Before enhancement with contrast demonstrating a large irregular lucent mass compressing the fourth ventricle. *b* After contrast enhancement, the lesion is more evident. Note lucent zones in the medial portion of the tumor.

Fig. 4. Small acoustic neurinoma 2 cm in size on the left, seen only following injection of contrast (arrows).

Table I. Cerebellopontine lesions

Acoustic neurinomas	27	Cysticercus cyst	1
Meningiomas	18	Chordoma	2
Trigeminal neurinomas	5	Metastatic	1
Epidermoid cyst	1	Pontine glioma (extension from)	4
Abscess	1	Cerebellar glioma (extension from)	3
Arachnoidal cyst	1	Aneurysm	2

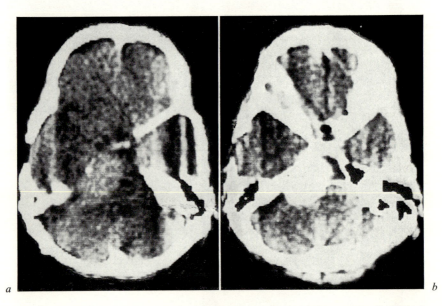

a   b

Fig.5. CPA meningioma on the left. *a* Before contrast enhancement. *b* Marked enhancement of the tumor after injection of contrast.

to exclude small intracanalicular tumors. Arteriography is performed when there is a definite positive scan of a CPA mass with atypical features or where a high degree of clinical suspicion exists in spite of the demonstration of normal internal auditory canals. Pneumography has been replaced by CT in the investigation of large CPA tumors. CT also has a definite value in the evaluation of the postoperative course, particularly in those cases where the tumor was only partially removed.

Both acoustic neurinomas and meningiomas enhance markedly following infusion of contrast. When these lesions are large in size, meningiomas en-

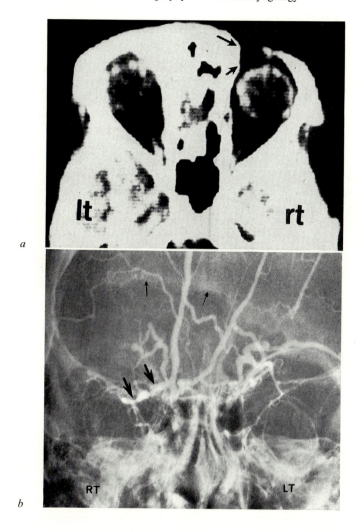

Fig.6. Right frontal mucocele. *a* CT demonstrating the destructive process in the superiomedial portion of the right orbit. *b* Orbital venogram showing the mass effect (large arrows) and the destructive process (small arrows).

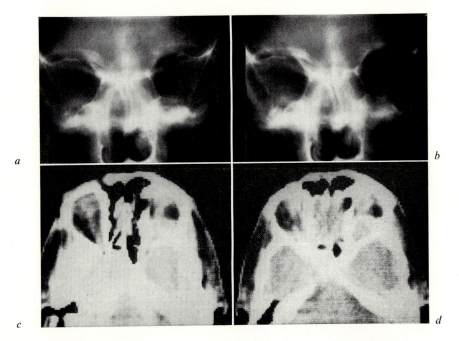

Fig. 7. Acute inflammatory process involving the ethmoidal area. *a* Conventional tomogram. *b* CT demonstrating the ethmoidal lesion extending into the orbital areas mainly on the right.

hance very homogeneously (fig. 5), whereas acoustic neurinomas may have central or peripheral lucent areas, which very well may represent necrotic portions of the tumor (fig. 3). Small meningiomas are rarely seen.

Trigeminal neuralgia may be the result of a pathological process for which the otorhinolaryngologist is first consulted. Symptoms may be produced by CPA tumors, benign or malignant processes confined to paranasal sinuses or extending into the intracranial cavity, orbital areas or pterygopalatine fossa [4, 5, 7, 8]. CT of these areas may offer additional information to the conventional methods for better assessment of those processes [fig. 6, 7].

New developments in CT imaging are rapidly taking place producing better resolution in the imaging, and displays which allows measurements of attenuation values in the different areas of interest.

The universal (body) scanner having a larger opening in the gantry, allowing the patients to be moved through, enables us to obtain better detail of axial sections of the base of the skull, face and neck. Placing the patients with the neck in hyperextension in either prone or supine position, coronal

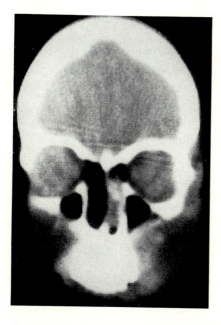

Fig.8. CT in the coronal plane demonstrating a malignant lesion involving the left nasal and ethmoidal area.

plane sections of the head can be obtained. This is facilitated if the CT unit is provided with a tilting gantry.

Coronal sections may be useful for the evaluation of abnormalities close to the base of the skull, sinuses, orbits and nasopharynx (fig. 8). Sections in different planes clarifies location, morphological characteristics, and volume of intracranial, orbital and facial structures. This information may be of significant importance for surgical and radiation therapy planning [5].

Improvements in contrast material opacification of the cerebrospinal pathways in order to demonstrate normal and abnormal subarachnoid space and ventricular morphology may soon become an accepted complimentary CT technique. Intrathecal injection of Metrizamide, a water contrast material, has demonstrated striking and encouraging results in preliminary investigations. The method appears to be helpful in the differentiation of intraaxial from extraaxial lesions and for documentation of intraventricular mass location. Also, the method may be helpful for diagnosis of arachnoiditis, ventricular obstruction, and impairment of cerebrospinal fluid circulation [5].

Summary

The value of computed tomography in ORL and its applications have been briefly discussed. Better soft tissue detail and its relationship to bony structures is obtained. At the present time this modality may be utilized as a screening test in some suspected cases or as an adjunct to conventional methods. With the technical refinements that are constantly being made, better diagnostic information will be obtained in CT scanning.

References

1   AMBROSE, J.: Computerized transverse axial scanning (tomography). 2. Clinical application. Br. J. Radiol. *46:* 1023–1047 (1973).
2   AMBROSE, J.: Computerized x-ray scanning of the brain. J. Neurosurg. *40:* 679–695 (1974).
3   BAKER, Ill., jr.; CAMPBELL, J.K.; HOUSER, O.W., *et al.:* Computer assisted tomography of the head. An early evaluation. Mayo Clin. Proc. *49:* 17–27 (1974).
4   GAWLER, J.; SANDERS, M.D.; BULL, J.W.D., *et al.:* Computer assisted tomography in orbital disease. Br. J. Ophthal. *48:* 471–587 (1974).
5   GONZALES, C.F.; GROSSMAN, C.B., and PALACIOS, E.: Computed brain and orbital tomography (Wiley, New York 1976).
6   HOUNSFIELD, G.B.: Computerized transverse axial scanning (tomography). 1. Description of system. Br. J. Radiol. *46:* 1015–1022 (1973).
7   LAMPERT, V.L.; ZELCH, J.V., and COHEN, D.N.: Computed tomography of the orbits. Radiology *113:* 351–354 (1974).
8   MAMOSE, K.K.; NEW, P.F.J.; GROVE, S.A., jr., and SCOTT, W.R.: The use of computed tomography in ophthamology. Radiology *115:* 361–368 (1975).
9   NEW, P.F.J.; SCOTT, W.R.; SCHNUR, J.A., *et al.:* Computed tomography with the EMI scanner in the diagnosis of primary and metastatic intracranial neoplasms. Radiology *114:* 75–87 (1975).
10 NEW, P.F.J.; SCOTT, W.R.; SCHNUR, J.A., *et al.:* Computerized axial tomography with the EMI scanner. Radiology *110:* 109–123 (1974).
11 NEW, P.F.J. and SCOTT, W.R.: Computed tomography of the brain and orbit (EMI scanning), pp. 194–198, 450–452 (Williams & Wilkins, Baltimore 1975).

ENRIQUE PALACIOS, MD, Department of Radiology, Loyola University of Chicago, 2160 South First Avenue, *Maywood, IL 60153* (USA)

Adv. Oto-Rhino-Laryng., vol. 24, pp. 9–20 (Karger, Basel 1978)

Value and Limits of
Computerized Axial Tomography in ORL

E. Schindler, A. Aulich and S. Wende[1]

Department of Neuroradiology (Head: Prof. Wende),
Neurosurgical University Hospital (Director: Prof. Schürmann), Mainz

In our neuroradiological department, computerized axial tomography (CT) is possible for 11 months now. In this period, we have examined with the EMI scanner the orbits and the adjacent structures of the paranasal sinuses of about 70 patients. A statistical evaluation of this material is not likely to be recommendable – thus we would prefer to demonstrate some CT findings and some radiographs in order to report our experience of value and limits of CT in ORL, and to raise some diagnostic questions, the discussion of which – in our opinion – could be interesting.

Figure 1a represents the computer tomograms of a squamous cell carcinoma. The lower section shows the tumor in the left maxillary ethmoid angle, spreading medially into posterior ethmoid cells and into the adjacent upper nasal meatus, whereas the sphenoid sinus seems not to be involved. Growing upwards and laterally the neoplasm has destroyed the medial orbital wall, invading the orbit and causing protrusion of the left bulb. The upper section reveals that the tumor has occupied almost completely the left ethmoid sinus. Comparing these CT findings with the pathologic changes visible on the tomograms (fig. 1b)[2] we cannot find an essential discrepancy; our EMI scanner, of course, cannot visualize the marked tumor expansion in the inferior parts of the facial region: maxillary sinus, nasal space on the left, palate, choana, pterygoid maxillary fossa.

CT of the next case (fig. 2a) yielded a mass in the left ethmoid sinus; a bone defect or a tumor invasion of the orbit is not to be seen. The axial tomogram (fig. 2b), however, shows distinctly that the tumor has destroyed

---

[1] Supported by the Deutsche Forschungsgemeinschaft.

[2] All the conventional tomograms of this paper are turned leftside-right for better comparison with the computer tomograms.

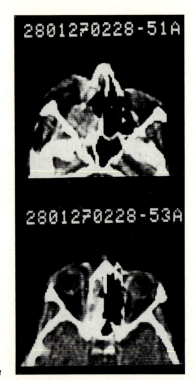

1 a

Fig. 1. Tumor in the left maxillary ethmoid angle. *a* CT. Tumor invasion of the orbit (causing exophthalmus) and the ethmoid on the left. *b* Conventional tomography. Extensive tumor spreading into the paranasal sinuses and the adjacent structures on the left. Squamous cell carcinoma.

the papyraceous plate, thus orbital involvement was to be surmised. In fact, the surgeon found a carcinoma of the ethmoid spreading into the medial part of the left orbit.

On the other hand, in the case represented in figure 3 CT gave better information than conventional tomography. A mass in the right nasolacrimal duct could be found by EMI scanning (fig. 3a), whereas the tomogram (fig. 3b) does not show any pathologic change at all. Operation and histology yielded a carcinoma which had not yet affected the adjacent bony walls, thus the tomogram seems quite normal.

The distinction by CT between malignant and benign space-occupying lesions and inflammatory changes is sometimes difficult. In figure 4a the CT section shows a high density region within the widened left ethmoid sinus, a bone defect of the medial orbital wall is not to be seen; the left bulb is slightly abducted. Based on CT alone, one cannot exclude an early stage of a malignant tumor, but the tomograms (fig. 4b) show the typical bulging of the papyraceous plate into the orbit which indicates a benign space-occupying lesion. A mucocele was found.

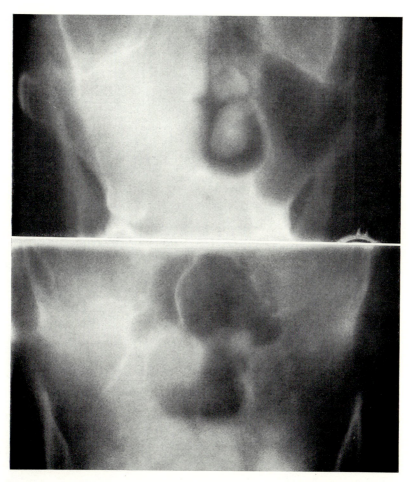

1b

Figure 5a shows the computer tomograms of a huge recurrent giant cell tumor which involves the left zygomaticoorbital region, almost the whole orbital floor and the lateral retrobulbar space, thus causing exophthalmus. The tumor has grown posteriorly into the temporal fossa, considerably destroying the bone. The tumor extent in the facial region is visualized also by tomography (fig. 5b), which reveals a tumor spreading into the right infraorbital region as well. Only CT, however, indicated a very unfavorable expansion (fig. 5c) – this is the intracranial tumor invasion. We have to assume this because of the well-defined higher density region (after enhance-

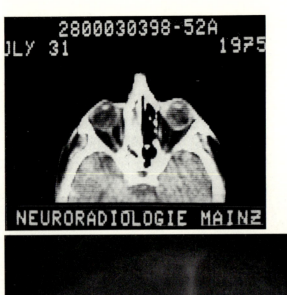

a

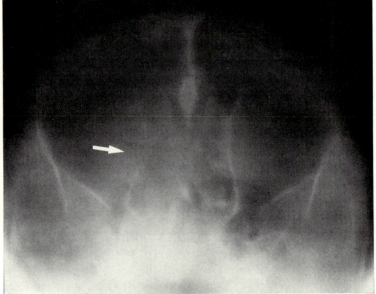

b

Fig. 2. Tumor in the ethmoid sinus. *a* CT. A tumor invasion of the orbit is not visible. *b* Axial tomography. Bone defect of the left papyraceous plate indicating tumor extent into the orbit. Solid carcinoma of the ethmoid.

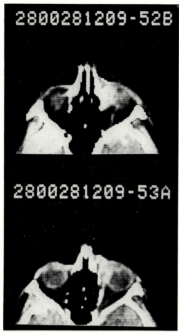

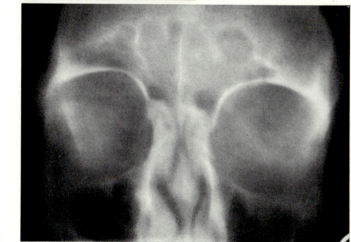

Fig. 3. a CT. Well-defined mass localized medially of the right bulb. *b* Conventional tomography. No pathologic changes visible. Carcinoma of the right nasolacrimal duct.

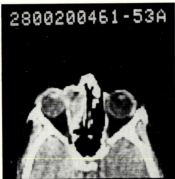

a

b

Fig.4. a CT. High-density region in the widened left ethmoid sinus; slight abduction of the left bulb. *b* Conventional tomography. Marked bulging of the left papyraceous plate into the orbit; no bone destruction. Mucocele.

ment) in the left medial cranial fossa, which has the same absorption values as found in the facial parts of the tumor, and which is surrounded by a lower density zone corresponding to local edema.

Concerning CT in cerebellopontine angle tumors, two cases shall be demonstrated. In the first case the positive contrast medium cisternogram (fig. 6a) shows a clearly outlined mass which is not visible at all in the EMI scan (fig. 6b), not even after intravenous injection of Conray; there are Pantopaque droplets in the basal cisterns. In the second case the cerebellopontine angle tumor, proved by Pantopaque cisternography (fig. 7a), is distinctly visualized by CT after contrast medium enhancement (fig. 7b); the fourth ventricle is shifted to the left. An acoustic neuroma, bulging only slightly into the cistern, was found in the first case, whereas figure 7 is a representation of a neuroma of about 35 mm in size, occupying completely the cerebellopontine angle. The difference in the CT findings of these cases mainly is due to the well-known fact that a tumor has to have a certain size to be shown by computer tomography. If this size is reached, however, Pantopaque cisternography or pneumoencephalography are not needed to diagnose a cerebellopontine angle tumor in most cases.

In tumors, particularly in the ORL region, the radiologist – using any X-ray method – generally is facing the following questions:

Localization of the tumor. Direction of the tumor growth. Reaction pattern of the tissue – particularly the bone tissue – which is surrounding the tumor. X-ray absorption value of the tumor tissue.

A specific tumor diagnosis based exclusively on radiological findings will be possible only in a very few cases.

Summarizing the limits of CT in ORL with regard to these questions we have to stress that the technical evolution of CT has just begun and will be essentially advanced within a foreseeable space of time. Furthermore, we would like to point out some of the problems to which radiologists will have to get down to contribute their medical part – besides the technical one – to the expansion of the diagnostic field of CT.

The *localization of a tumor* can be shown by CT only if this tumor is situated in an area which can be reached by the scanning X-ray. Our scanner is able to draw regions superior to the orbital floors. Maxillary sinus, choana, nasopharynx as well as pterygoid maxillary fossa are outside the reach of the EMI scanner, which is working with a rubber cap and a water-containing box around the patient's head. There are already developed scanners which do not need this apparatus; they will considerably extend the diagnostic possibilities of CT in ORL.

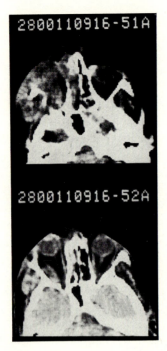

5 a

The same restriction as mentioned above applies to the demonstration of the *direction of the tumor growth:* We cannot make sure by CT whether a tumor is spreading into inferior parts of the face or not. We think, however, that a prognostically very important question can be answered by CT, i.e. whether a tumor has invaded the intracranial space or not. In most such cases the different absorption values – corresponding to the higher density of tumor tissue or to the less absorbing brain edema surrounding the tumor – can be measured and indicated by the computer.

As far as the *reaction pattern of the tumor-surrounding tissue* is concerned, we mean that conventional tomography shows earlier and more exactly that a tumor has destroyed bony walls invading neighboring areas. On a tomogram we can see the pathologic bone structures caused by expansive tumor growth or by infiltrating spreading of a malignant neoplasm. These changes are not visualized by CT, but there is hope that technical progress and investigation in particular of CT findings in bone changes will bring forth important results.

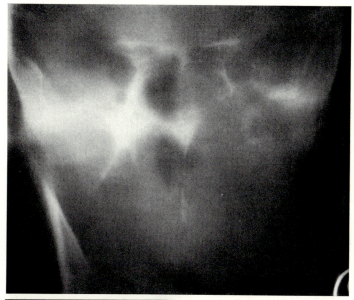

5 b

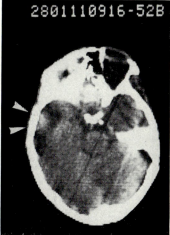

5 c

Fig.5. a CT of superior facial areas. Huge mass on the left involving the zygomatico-orbital region, spreading posteriorly into the temporal fossa (distinct bone destruction) and medially into the lateral retrobulbar space, causing exophthalmus. *b* Conventional tomography. Tumor expansion also into the right infraorbital region (extensive bone defects on the right because of surgical intervention). *c* CT of the intracranial space. High-density region in the left medial cranial fossa surrounded by a lower density zone, indicating intracranial tumor invasion. Giant cell tumor.

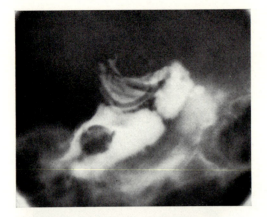

a

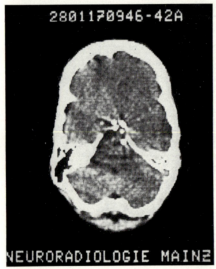

b

Fig.6. Cerebellopontine angle tumor on the right. *a* Pantopaque cisternography. The tumor is clearly outlined. *b* CT (after enhancement). The tumor is not visible. Acoustic neuroma.

The most progressive results, however, we can expect from an intensive and systematic study of the *X-ray absorption values* of different tumors in CT – this research could lead to a differential diagnosis of tumors by means of X-rays only. There is no doubt that just CT and density measurement is the only way to get there.

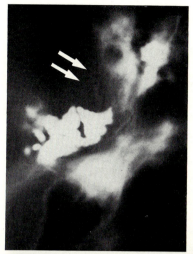

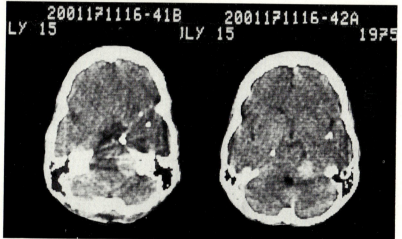

Fig. 7 Cerebellopontine angle tumor on the right. *a* Pantopaque cisternography. Large mass in the cerebellopontine angle cistern. *b* CT (after enhancement). The tumor is distinctly visualized; the 4th ventricle is shifted to the left. Acoustic neuroma.

Obviously, there are lots of problems still unsolved, and in a certain way we are just at the beginning of CT in ORL. We find ourselves on the border of a highly interesting scientific field, whose exploration will be practicable only by means of combination and correlation of clinical and conventional radiological findings with the results of computerized axial tomography.

Summary

The CT findings in some selected cases presenting lesions of the paranasal sinuses and the orbits are compared with the conventional tomograms. Referring to these examples, our experience of value and limits of CT in ORL is reported. Furthermore, a few remarks to CT in cerebellopontine angle tumors are given. Finally, there are pointed out some general considerations concerning radiodiagnostic questions in tumors of the ORL region.

References

NEW, P.F.J. and SCOTT, W.R.: Computed tomography of the brain and orbit (EMI scanning) (Williams & Wilkins, Baltimore 1975).

REISNER, K. and GOSEPATH, J.: Schädeltomographie (Thieme, Stuttgart 1973).

VALVASSORI, G.E.: The abnormal internal auditory canal: the diagnosis of acoustic neuroma. Radiology *92:* 449–459 (1969).

WUSTROW, F.: Die Tumoren des Gesichtsschädels (Urban & Schwarzenberg, München 1965).

Dr. E. SCHINDLER, Department of Neuroradiology, Neurosurgical University Hospital, Langenbeckstrasse 1, *D–6500 Mainz* (FRG)

Adv. in Oto-Rhino-Laryng., vol. 24, pp. 21–31 (Karger, Basel 1978)

Computerized Scanning in Otorhinolaryngology

Barbara L. Carter, Steven B. Hammerschlag
and Samuel M. Wolpert

Department of Radiology, Division of Neuroradiology,
Tufts-New England Medical Center, Boston, Mass.

Computed whole body scanning, evolving from the original work of
Hounsfield [8,9], has introduced a new era in otorhinolaryngology by
making significant contributions to both the diagnosis and the care of the
patient with disease of the head and neck area [5–7]. Examples of the use
of this technique will be demonstrated and the advantages discussed.

Method

The scans were obtained with the Ohio-Nuclear Delta Whole Body
Scanner with dual beam 13 mm collimation. The angle of the scanning plane
and total number of scan pairs varied with the region studied. Initially,
images were recorded on Polaroid film and subsequently on X-ray film using
the Deltamat Recorder. At least two different settings were used for each
image to obtain maximum detail of bone, soft tissue and air-containing
structures. A wide window of 800–3,000 Delta units (also referred to as
EMI units, which are equal to one half the Delta units, or as Hounsfield
numbers) yielded the best visualization of bone and air-containing structures
whereas a narrow window of 100–800 Delta units was utilized for greater
contrast and thus better soft tissue detail. A high centering of 100–200 Delta
units was best for studying bone, a lower centering of 10–30 units for soft
tissue structures. Contrast enhancement was used when indicated [1].

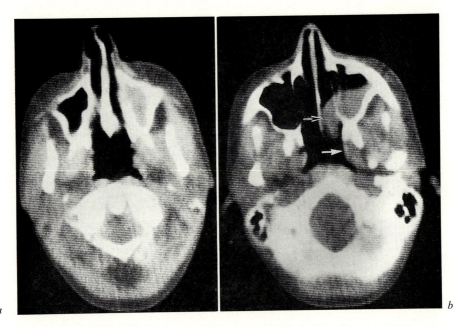

a   *b*

Fig. 1. a This woman was suspected of having carcinoma and was found to have an opaque left maxillary antrum. *b* A more cephalic scan reveals an antral-choanal polyp (black arrow) projecting back toward the nasopharynx. There is slight flattening of the lateral wall (white arrow) of the nasopharynx but the soft tissues are otherwise normal.

Case Material

Several patients are presented to demonstrate the usefulness of computed tomography (CT) scanning in the following areas: (1) paranasal sinuses, (fig. 1–3), (2) the nasopharynx (fig. 4), (3) salivary glands (fig. 5, 6), (4) soft tissue of the neck (fig. 7, 8), and (5) petrous bone (fig. 9, 10).

Discussion

The radiological evaluation of disease involving primarily soft tissues of the head and neck areas has often required the use of tomography, angiography, radionuclide scanning and other special techniques. These, however, have not yielded adequate visualization of the total area of involvement. This is now possible with CT scanning [11], a significant advancement in the

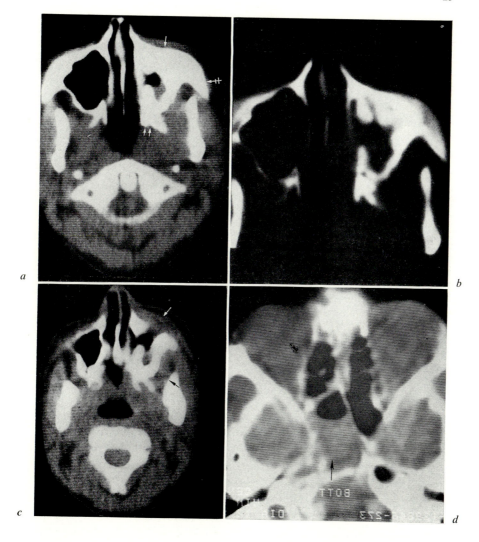

Fig. 2. This man has chronic sinusitis due to pseudomonas infection superimposed on leukemic infiltration of the sinus. Extensive hyperostosis (a) involves all the walls of the maxillary sinus (single arrow), the zygoma (crossed arrow) and the pterygoid plates (double arrows). This is better appreciated using higher centering for bone detail (b). There is considerable soft tissue involvement (c) anteriorly (white arrow) and laterally (black arrow) between the maxillary sinus and ramus of the mandible. The patient later returned with right retro-orbital pain with a presumptive diagnosis of leukemic infiltration of the orbit or of retrobulbar hematoma. CT scan (d) reveals an opaque right sphenoid sinus (black arrow), presumably sinusitis, which cleared.

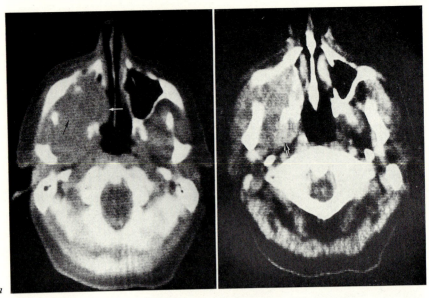

a

Fig. 3. a Extensive destruction of the medial (white arrow), posterolateral (black arrow) and anterior walls of the right maxillary sinus is due to tumor. *b* Note the large soft tissue extension of the tumor (black arrow), clearly seen on this second scan taken at a lower level with a relatively narrow window.

diagnosis and treatment of patients. We have presented several examples of these for the region of the sinuses, nasopharynx, salivary glands, neck and petrous bone. The transverse plane adds a new dimension to the coronal and sagittal planes; soft tissue detail is better than that obtained with any other modality, yet bone detail is also remarkably good. For instance, it is possible to identify the ossicular chain and the ostium of the cochlear aqueduct with the proper scanning plane and window settings [3]. In our series, unsuspected lesions have been discovered, suspect tumors more clearly defined, and the total extent of disease more precisely determined than has heretofore been possible. This is of particular importance to the radiotherapist in planning treatment portals [4, 10] and to the oncologist in determining response of tumor to treatment. The role of angiography is still important in certain lesions such as angiofibromas, chemodectomas, AVMs, etc. to confirm the diagnosis and at times to aid in treatment by embolization.

Inflammatory and neoplastic involvement of the paranasal sinuses have traditionally been studied by plain radiographs and tomography. CT scanning has proven useful [12] in delineating benign polypoid disease (fig. 1), in

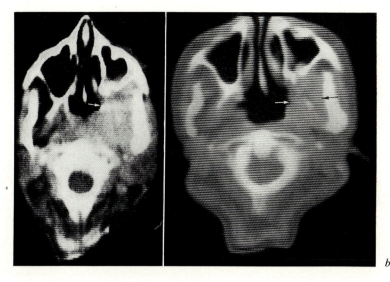

a   b

Fig. 4. A large tumor of the nasopharynx (a) with destruction of the pterygoid plates (white arrow) extends into the maxillary sinus and is involving all of the soft tissues between the maxillary sinus and the mandible. The patient improved with radiation therapy but still had difficulty opening her mouth. A follow-up CT scan (b) reveals residual tumor or indurated tissue (arrows) on the left side, involving the pterygoid muscles.

demonstrating extension of inflammatory disease outside the sinuses (fig. 2), and in defining the total extent of malignant disease (fig. 3). Nasopharyngeal tumors may be so large as to present some distance from the site of origin and thus be mistaken for a different type of lesion. A patient (fig. 4) was originally found to have an opaque maxillary sinus. This was biopsied and proved to be malignant. It was considered to be a carcinoma of the maxillary sinus until the CT scan revealed the major portion of the tumor to be in the nasopharynx. The patient improved with radiation therapy, but was unable to open her mouth even after completion of her treatments. Abnormal tissue representing either residual tumor or indurated scar tissue was found in the region of the pterygoid muscles (fig. 4b). Small tumors limited to the nasal cavity or nasopharynx may not be visible on plain film studies or hypocycloidal tomography but are apparent by CT scanning. This has on several occasions been the only means of establishing the diagnosis by documenting the area to be biopsied. Tumors of the salivary glands are usually outlined by sialography. When a soft tissue mass is close to the surface of a gland, it may be difficult to determine whether it is within or just outside the gland. The normal parotid

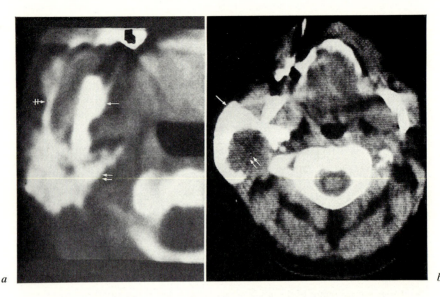

a   *b*

Fig. 5. a A normal CT scan taken after a right parotid sialogram shows the deep lobe of the parotid gland (double arrows) just behind the mandible (single arrow) with Stensen's duct (crossed arrow) anterior to the parotid gland. *b* A mixed tumor (double arrow) of the right parotid gland (single arrow) is deep within the gland, clearly shown by CT scanning.

(fig. 5a) is compared to a gland containing a tumor (fig. 5b). Although large tumors are visible to the naked eye, the total extent of the tumor is best determined by CT scan (fig. 6) allowing for precise localization and planning of radiation therapy portals.

Soft tissue masses in the neck are often palpable in a normal sized person, but a muscular or obese individual may be difficult to examine. Many of these lesions such as metastatic nodes, lymphoma, branchial cleft cysts (fig. 7), tumors deep-seated within the neck, associated with but extending beyond the cervical spine [5], carotid body tumors (fig. 8), thyroid nodules and lesions of the larynx and pharynx are sharply defined by CT scan. This has proven to be of particular value to the surgeon in localizing relatively small tumors such as parathyroid adenomas [2].

Finally, lesions of the base of the skull are visible by CT scanning [5] yielding as much information and sometimes more than plain film studies and tomography. The diagnoses of acoustic neuromas, meningiomas around the skull base (and elsewhere within the skull), tumors within and around the sella and orbit have been well documented. Other disease entitites involving

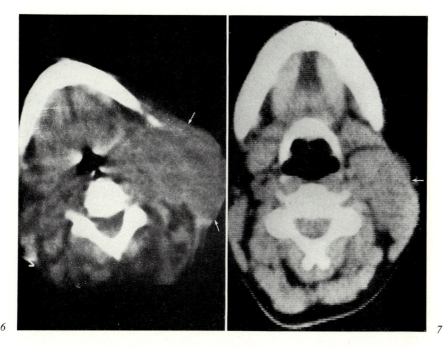

6   7

Fig.6. A very large parotid gland tumor (arrows) demonstrated by CT scanning is seen to extend deep to the cervical spine. Several scans were obtained to determine the total extent of the tumor.

Fig.7. A branchial cleft cyst (arrow) on the left side of the neck is sharply defined. Whereas most cystic lesions have relatively low absorption coefficients, this appears somewhat dense possibly related to its fluid content (discarded before it could be analyzed).

the base of the skull have been studied, including those within the petrous bone as demonstrated in figures 9 and 10. The results are equal to that achieved by a combination of other studies which are more costly and require hospitalization (angiography, pneumoencephalography). The patient in figure 9 has had a previous exploratory operation of the middle cranial fossa on the right side for a mass which was biopsied and reported as cholesteatoma. AP and lateral tomograms of the ear obtained on the present hospitalization revealed findings typical of acquired cholesteatoma. However, in view of her previous surgical findings with the presumptive diagnosis of a primary intracranial lesion, it was important to determine the presence of any residual intracranial disease. A CT scan was done which demonstrated the total extent of bone involvement (correlating well with the polytome studies obtained in the AP, lateral and base projections) and ruled out any intracranial disease.

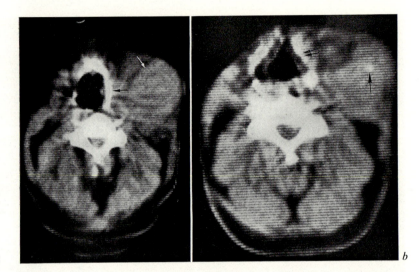

a   *b*

Fig. 8. a A large submandibular mass (white arrow) lateral to the hyoid bone (black arrow) is clearly seen. *b* The second scan is taken at the upper level of the thyroid cartilage (double arrow). Contrast enhancement was not done, but calcification (single arrow) is visible. The mass proved to be a chemodectoma involving the carotid body.

The need for any further invasive procedures was eliminated. The last operation was thus confined to her tympanic cavity.

Another patient (fig. 10) was found by clinical examination to have a vascular tumor of her left ear. At the time of operation by mastoid approach, the surgeon encountered a gush of blood from the operative site and discontinued his procedure. Subsequent tomograms confirmed the presence of a tumor within the tympanic cavity and mastoid area, but there was no enlargement or destruction of the jugular fossa and a vascular tumor was not identified by angiography. A CT scan also demonstrated opacification of the tympanic cavity and mastoid air cells, but no evidence of bone destruction. In addition, a more cephalic scan (not shown) revealed that the previous operative defect extended posterior directly into the sigmoid sinus, thus explaining the 'gush of blood' at the time of the original operation. All findings including the CT scan were consistent with the presence of a glomus tympanicum which was proven by subsequent surgery.

The bone destruction around the jugular bulb due to a glomus jugulare tumor is apt to be more extensive than with a glomus tympanicum but very permeative and difficult to demonstrate. Multiple projections by polytomo-

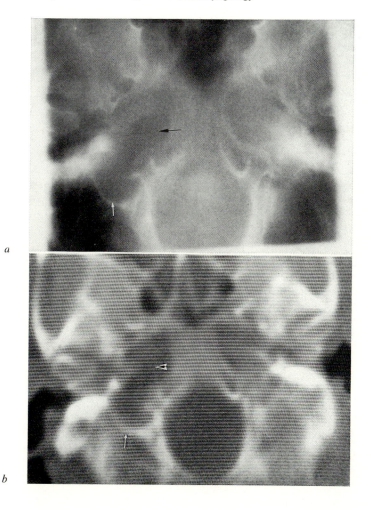

a

b

Fig.9. A hypocycloidal tomogram (a) and a CT scan (b) of the base of the skull in a patient with extensive destruction of the petrous bone by cholesteatoma. The petrous apex (black arrow) on the right side has been partially destroyed, the area of involvement extending back to the jugular fossa (white arrow). The bone detail of the CT scan, though not quite as sharp as the polytome, is sufficiently clear to be diagnostic. (The CT scan was necessary to rule out recurrent intracranial extension.)

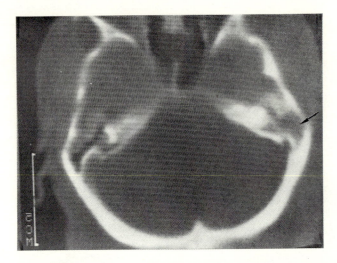

Fig. 10. A soft tissue mass (arrow) within the left tympanic cavity and mastoid air cells had no evidence of bone destruction on CT scan other than a previous operative defect opposite the sigmoid sinus. Multiple projections by polytomography confirmed the diffuse soft tissue opacity throughout the left ear, without evidence of bone destruction. The diagnosis of glomus tympanicum was confirmed at surgery.

graphy may thus be necessary to determine total extent of the disease prior to biopsy and treatment. CT scanning appears to give comparable information about extent of bone destruction (especially if there is some overlap of the scans) and has the added benefit of demonstrating extension of tumor into the adjacent soft tissue area.

Conclusion

CT scanning in the head and neck area has proven to be a very valuable tool in the diagnosis and treatment of disease. Good bone detail can be obtained, large and small soft tissue tumors identified. Examples of this have been illustrated. Considerable experience with this new modality must be accumulated to determine its future role in otorhinolaryngology. Our early experience is encouraging. In many cases, it appears to be the study of choice, often eliminating the need for other time-consuming and, sometimes, invasive procedures.

Acknowledgment

The authors wish to express their appreciation to PATRICIA JAYSON for her assistance in the organization of this paper.

References

1   CARTER, B.L. and IGNATOW, S.: Neck and mediastinal angiography by CT Scan. Radiology *122:* 515–516 (1977).
2   CARTER, B.L. and IGNATOW, S.: CT scanning of parathyroid tumors (in preparation).
3   CARTER, B.L.; MOREHEAD, J.; WOLPERT, S.M.; HAMMERSCHLAG, S.B.; GRIFFITHS, H.J., and KAHN, P.C.: Cross-sectional anatomy. Computed tomography and ultrasound correlation (Appleton-Century-Crofts, New York, 1977).
4   CHERNAK, E.S.; RODRIQUEZ-ANTUNEZ, A.; JELDEN, G.L.; DHALIEVAL, R., and LARIK, P.S.: The use of computed tomography for radiation therapy treatment planning. Radiology *117:* 613–614 (1975).
5   HAMMERSCHLAG, S.B.; WOLPERT, S.M., and CARTER, B.L.: Computed tomography of the skull base. J. Comput. Assist. Tomography *1:* 75–80 (1977).
6   HAMMERSCHLAG, S.B.; WOLPERT, S.M., and CARTER, B.L.: Computed tomography of the spinal canal. Radiology *121:* 361–367 (1976).
7   HAMMERSCHLAG, S.B.; WOLPERT, S.M., and CARTER, B.L.: Computed coronal tomography. Radiology *120:* 219–220 (1976).
8   HOUNSFIELD, G.N.: Computerized transverse axial scanning. Br.J.Radiol. *46:* 1016–1022 (1973).
9   HOUNSFIELD, G.N.: Picture quality of computed tomography. Am.J.Roentg. *127:* 3–9 (1976).
10 MUNZENRIDER, J.E.; PILEPICH, M.; RENE-FERRERO, J.B.; TCHAKAROVA, I., and CARTER, B.L.: Use of body scanner in radiotherapy treatment planning (submitted for publication).
11 SADAMOTO, K.: The cranio-cervical computed tomography developed in Japan and its vertical axial scanning. E120 Jō kō Medical-Image Technology and Information Display *8:10 (94):* 41–52 (1976).
12 WORTZMAN, G. and HOLGATE, R.C.: Special radiological techniques in maxillary sinus disease. Otolar.Clins N. Am. *9:* 117–133 (1976).

B.L.CARTER, MD, Department of Radiology, 171 Harrison Avenue, *Boston, MA 02111* (USA)

Adv. Oto-Rhino-Laryng., vol. 24, pp. 32–33 (Karger, Basel 1978)

Acoustic Neuroma Diagnosis by CT: Analysis and Evaluation of Findings

KENNETH R. DAVIS, STEPHEN W. PARKER and ALFRED WEBER

Departments of Radiology and Neurology, Massachusetts General Hospital, and Departments of Radiology and Neurology, Massachusetts Eye & Ear Infirmary, Boston, Mass.

Acoustic neuromas are composed of Schwann cells that originate from and envelope the axons of the eighth nerve, particularly the vestibular branch. Prior to the availability of computed tomography (CT), invasive studies such as pneumoencephalography, pantopaque cisternography, and occasionally angiography were utilized in various combinations (following plain films and laminagrams) for radiographic detection and estimation of the size of an acoustic neuroma. The radiologic approach has changed in that CT is now obtained prior to invasive studies, which frequently obviates the necessity of the latter. The incidence of false-negative CT scans, and comparison of CT and surgical size of the lesion were evaluated retrospectively from surgically proven cases.

Review of CT scans in 52 consecutive patients with surgically excised acoustic neuromas revealed positive scans in 39 (75%) following contrast enhancement, with 13 (25%) false-negative scans (fig. 1, 2). The positive scans were evaluated to assess the predictive value in determining the size of the lesion, since the operative approach varies according to the maximal diameter. The CT-surgical correlation indicated uniform CT underestimation of size in all but one case. This is likely due to limited visualization during surgery and also to partial volume effect. In order to overcome this potential CT limitation, it is desirable to use thin (8 mm or less) and often overlapping sections through the cerebellopontine angle region so that the equator of the tumor is fully included and completely fills the largest possible number of picture elements in the section.

K.R. DAVIS, MD, Department of Radiology, Massachusetts General Hospital, *Boston, MA 02114* (USA)

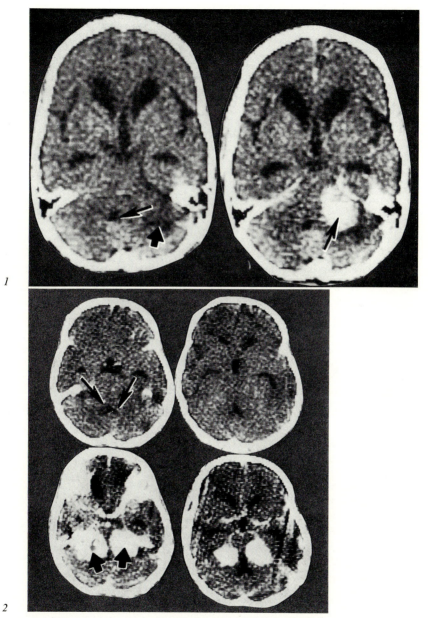

Fig.1. Acoustic neuroma with positive plain and positive CE scan. Left: Plain study. Displacement of fourth ventricle to the left (→). Low absorption abnormality in the right cerebellopontine angle (➡). Right: CE-CT. High absorption abnormality in right cerebellopontine angle (→) with low absorption area of edema at posterior lateral aspect.

Fig.2. Bilateral acoustic neuromas in neurofibromatosis. Top: Plain CT. Bilateral compression of fourth ventricle (→). Bottom: CE-CT scan. Bilateral neuromas (➡).

Adv. Oto-Rhino-Laryng., vol. 24, pp. 34–38 (Karger, Basel 1978)

Computed Tomography of the Postoperative Acoustic Neuroma

LARISSA T. BILANIUK and ROBERT A. ZIMMERMAN

Department of Radiology, Hospital of the University of Pennsylvania, Philadelphia, Pa.

Computed tomography (CT) is a highly accurate noninvasive method for both preoperative [1] and postoperative evaluation of cerebellopontine angle lesions. In a review of 4,000 consecutive CT scans over a 17-month period at the Hospital of the University of Pennsylvania, 23 patients were examined following surgery for acoustic neuromas (table I). Immediate post-

Table I. Frequency of early and late postoperative changes following surgery for acoustic neuromas

Computed tomographic findings	Number of cases
I. Immediately after surgery	
Residual tumor	2
Complications	
Infarction	1
Hematoma	1
Infection	1
Operative changes only	6
Total patients	11
II. Long term follow-up	
Tumor, residual or recurrent	5
Sequelae	
Cyst	1
Postoperative encephalomalacia	9
Hydrocephalus	4
Total patients	16[1]

[1] Four patients from category I are also included in category II; 3 patients in category II had more than one sequela.

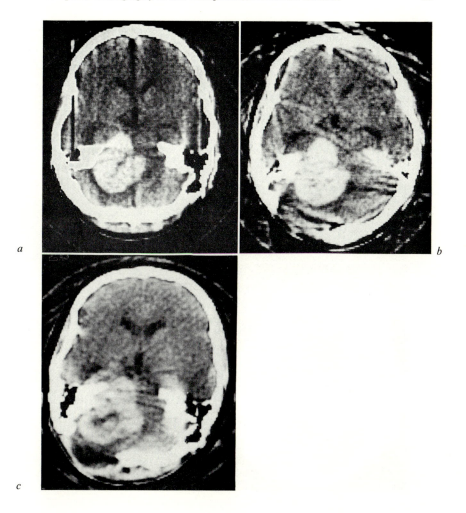

a

b

c

Fig. 1. Residual tumor. 23-year-old male with progressive hearing loss, tinnitus, vertigo, and ataxia. Paralysis of the right fifth, sixth, seventh, and eighth cranial nerves. *a* Postcontrast material injection CT scan demonstrates a large left cerebellopontine angle acoustic neuroma and hydrocephalus. *b* Second CT scan following what was stated to be a 60% resection shows no significant change and persistent hydrocephalus. *c* The third CT scan following what was stated to be a 90% resection shows no topographical change, but a central defect.

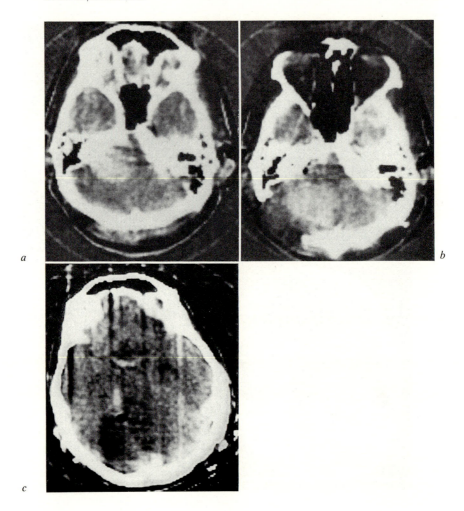

Fig. 2. Infarction. 55-year-old male presented with left hearing loss. *a* Preoperative scan with contrast material injection shows a left cerebellopontine angle acoustic neuroma. *b* 10 days following resection, the patient's condition deteriorated and CT scan *without contrast* material injection shows hemorrhagic infarction of the left cerebellar hemisphere. *c* Follow-up CT scan 1 week later shows cavitation under pressure of the infarcted area.

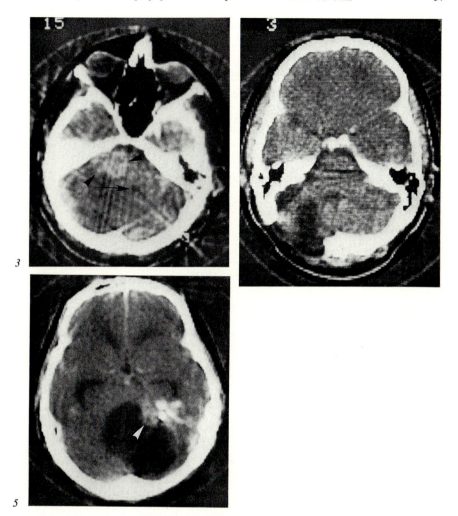

Fig. 3. Hematoma. 60-year-old male developed brain stem signs 10 days after resection of a large left acoustic neuroma. An emergency CT scan reveals a hematoma (arrowhead) in the brain stem and cerebellopontine angle cistern. The fourth ventricle (arrow) is compressed and displaced to the right.

Fig. 4. Postoperative encephalomalacia. 48-year-old male 6 years after resection of left acoustic neuroma with dizziness and weakness. There is no recurrence. Postoperative changes consisting of cerebellar encephalomalacia and enlargement of the cerebellopontine angle cistern are shown.

Fig. 5. Residual tumor with arachnoid cyst. 66-year-old male 14 years after subtotal resection of right acoustic neuroma developed right facial weakness and ataxia. CT scan shows a large arachnoid cyst arising from residual right acoustic neuroma (arrowhead).

operative period (table I): CT detects and delineates residual tumor (fig. 1) as well as complications such as infarction [2] (fig. 2), hematoma [3] (fig. 3), and infection [4].

Long-term postoperative evaluation (table I): CT can differentiate post-surgical changes, such as postoperative encephalomalacia (fig. 4) from recurrent or residual tumor (fig. 5). Sequelae of previous surgery such as arachnoid cysts and hydrocephalus are well demonstrated.

CT is effective and accurate in the differential diagnosis of postoperative problems and thus leads to appropriate therapeutic measures. The ease, speed, and noninvasiveness of the technique allow precise follow-up.

References

1   BAKER, H. L. and HOUSER, O. W.: Computed tomography in the diagnosis of posterior fossa lesions. Radiol. Clins N. Am. *14:* 129–147 (1976).
3   DAVIS, K. R.; TAVERAS, J. M.; NEW, P. E. J.; SCHNUR, J. A., and ROBERSON, G. H.: Cerebral infarction diagnosis by computerized tomography. Am. J. Roentg. *124:* 643–660 (1975).
2   SCOTT, W. R.; NEW, P. F.; DAVIS, K. R., and SCHNUR, J. A.: Computerized axial tomography of intracerebral and intraventricular hemorrhage. Radiology *112:* 73–80 (1974).
4   ZIMMERMAN, R. A.; PATEL, S., and BILANIUK, L. T.: Demonstration of purulent bacterial intracranial infections by computed tomography. Am. J. Roentg. *127:* 155–165 (1976).

Dr. L. T. BILANIUK, Department of Radiology, Hospital of the University of Pennsylvania, 3400 Spruce Street, *Philadelphia, PA 19104* (USA)

Adv. Oto-Rhino-Laryng., vol. 24, pp. 39–41 (Karger, Basel 1978)

Computed Tomography of Tumors of the Sphenoid Sinus and Bone

Robert A. Zimmerman and Larissa T. Bilaniuk

Department of Radiology, Hospital of the University of Pennsylvania, Philadelphia, Pa.

In a series of 4,000 consecutive CT scans, there were 33 cases of tumors that arose in or involved the sphenoid sinus or bone. These consisted of primary and secondary sphenoid tumors and tumors that extended from other paranasal sinuses, nasopharynx, or the brain.

CT accurately delineates the sphenoid sinus and bone, and shows their relationship to the rest of the cranial base, cranial fossa, and the orbits. The multiple adjacent sections obtained enable three-dimensional reconstruction.

Important information supplied by CT for differential diagnosis is density and topography of a lesion, and evidence of bony destruction. Detection of

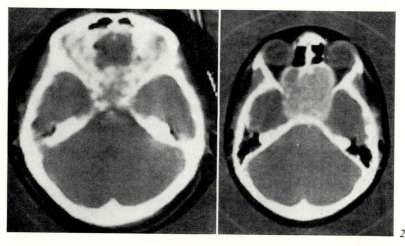

1
2

Fig. 1. Chondrosarcoma of the sphenoid. 53-year-old female with coma and history of therapy for lymphosarcoma of the neck 4 years ago. CT scan shows an enlarged opacified sphenoid sinus with stippled calcifications.

Fig. 2. Ossifying fibroma of the sphenoid. 14-year-old male with sudden left blindness. CT scan shows a diffusely dense lesion that expands the sphenoid bone.

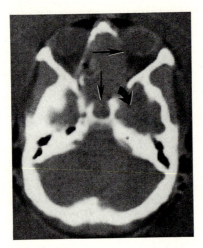

Fig. 3. Lymphoma. 33-year-old male with right proptosis. CT scan demonstrates poorly marginated lesion with bone destruction (arrows). The tumor involves sphenoid sinus, ethmoid sinuses, nasopharynx, nasal cavity, and the right orbit. There is also extension into the right cavernous sinus and middle cranial fossa (curved arrow).

calcification and its distribution within a lesion helps in etiologic diagnosis. Presence of stippled calcifications within a sphenoid mass is consistent with a tumor of cartilaginous origin (fig. 1) [1]. A diffusely dense lesion which expands the sphenoid sinus and is sharply marginated most often is due to osteoma [2], ossifying fibroma [3] (fig. 2), or fibrous dysplasia [4, 5]. Presence of a mass with bony destruction often indicates a malignant process (fig. 3) [6, 7]. This is best delineated by CT. Multidirectional tomography fails to show soft tissue invasion and the posterior extent.

References

1   MINAGI, H. and NEWTON, T. H.: Cartilaginous tumors of the base of the skull. Am. J. Roentg. *105:* 303–313 (1969).
2   CHILDREY, J. H.: Osteoma of the sinuses, the frontal and the sphenoid bone. Archs Otolar. *30:* 63–72 (1939).
3   MALCOMSON, K. G.: Clinical records ossifying fibroma of the sphenoid. J. Lar. Otol. *81:* 87–92 (1967).

4 WYLLIE, J.W.; KERN, E.B., and DJALILLIAN, M.: Isolated sphenoid sinus lesions. Laryngoscope *83:* 1252–1265 (1973).
5 SMITH, A.G. and ZAVALETA, A.: Osteoma, ossifying fibroma and fibrous dysplasia of facial and cranial bones. Archs Path. *54:* 507–527 (1952).
6 MILLER, W.E.; HOLMAN, C.B.; DOCKERTY, M.B., and DEVINE, K.D.: Roentgenologic manifestations of malignant tumors of the nasopharynx. Am.J.Roentg. *106:* 813–823 (1969).
7 FRAZELL, E.L. and LEWIS, J.S.: Cancer of the nasal cavity and accesory sinuses. Cancer *16:* 1293–1301 (1963).

R.A.ZIMMERMAN, MD, Department of Radiology, Hospital of the University of Pennsylvania, 3400 Spruce Street, *Philadelphia, PA 19104* (USA)

Adv. Oto-Rhino-Laryng., vol. 24, pp. 42–50 (Karger, Basel 1978)

Computed Tomography of the Paranasal Sinuses

Å. Forssell and B. Liliequist

Department of Neuroradiology (Director: B. Liliequist), University of Umeå, Umeå

In many diseases affecting the paranasal sinuses and its surrounding bone structures X-ray examination forms a necessary diagnostic procedure. Usually the conventional methods, i.e. plain film examination and tomography will give sufficient information about the nature and the extent of a lesion. However, in certain instances computer tomography may contribute further information.

The present study is intended to be merely a pilot investigation regarding the applicability of computer tomography in the investigation of diseases of the paranasal sinuses.

Technical Considerations

The examination of the paranasal sinuses with computer tomography presents certain difficulties due to the fact that the facial bones are inhomogenous and partly consist of thin bone plates surrounded by air. Hence, these structures show great variations in attenuation, which is reflected in the requirement of an extended range of EMI numbers displayed in the grey scale. In addition, the readings generally has to be displayed at more than one window level in order to make clear the relationship between bone structures and soft tissue.

In computer tomography as in the use of conventional X-ray techniques the choice of projection, depending on the structure to be investigated, is highly important. However, in the original EMI scanner variation in projection is limited due to the design of the headbox and its rubber cap, and structures below the base of the skull are mostly out of reach.

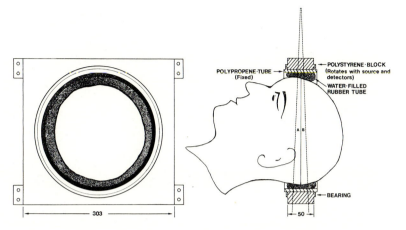

Fig. 1. The waterbox is substituted by a polystyrene block. The head of the patient is resting on a fixture-pillar and is further supported by a water-filled rubber tube.

To overcome these disadvantages WICKMAN suggested and developed a modification of the original headbox (fig. 1). Further technical details regarding the modification will be discussed in a later report [LILIEQUIST and WICKMAN, to be published].

Material and Method

The present series is selected among 300 examinations, the majority of which primarily referred to the brain and only a few to the paranasal sinuses. All the examinations but one were carried out with the original EMI scanner. A 160 × 160 matrix was used and the section thickness was 8 mm in three cases with maxillary carcinoma and 13 mm in the remaining cases. Pathological findings to be discussed below are carcinoma and fractures.

Results

Normal Anatomy

Valuable information concerning the soft tissue of the retropharyngeal space and the epipharynx may be obtained from sections of the nasopharynx (fig. 2). In appropriate sections details of the nasal cavity and the maxillary sinus may be identified (fig. 3). The important relationship between the orbit and the ethmoidal and the sphenoidal sinuses is well illustrated in figure 4.

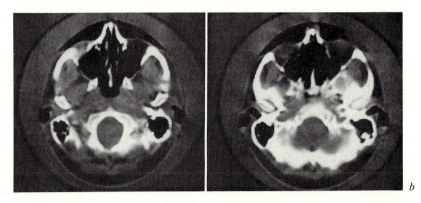

a   *b*

Fig. 2. Nasopharynx. *a* Part of the nasal cavity with the inferior conchae and the middle portion of the vomer. Behind the nasal cavity is the nasopharynx with the pterygoid processes on both sides. *b* The uppermost part of the nasopharynx with the posterior part of the vomer.

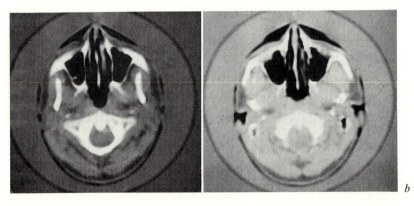

a   *b*

Fig. 3. Nasal cavity and maxillary sinus, examined with the modified scanner. *a* Details of the nasal cavity with the vomer and the inferior nasal concha. Both the medial and the lateral plate of the pterygoid process can be identified. *b* The middle nasal meatus with the maxillary hiatus.

Carcinoma

Three cases with malignant tumor of the paranasal sinuses have been investigated. In all three cases the tumors were anaplastic carcinomas, issuing from the maxillary sinus.

In the first case computer tomography revealed bone destruction in the anterior and the medial wall of the maxillary sinus. There was no sign of tumor in the ethmoidal cells, but the bottom of the orbit was considered

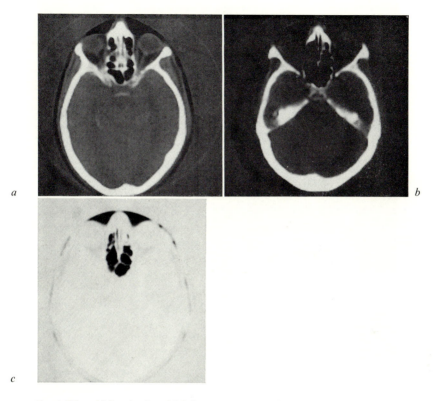

a

b

c

Fig. 4. Ethmoidal and sphenoidal sinuses. *a* Details of the sphenoid bone, for instance the anterior clinoid process, the dorsum sellae and the pituitary fossa as well as the optic canal are easily recognized. *b* The uppermost part of the nasal cavity with the perpendicular plate of the ethmoid bone. *c* By using a lower window level the very thin septa of the ethmoidal sinuses can be visualized.

to be involved (fig. 5). No additional information was supplied by linear tomography.

In the second case a Caldwell-Luc operation had been performed some months before the present examination. The operation was followed by radiological treatment. At computer tomography there was evidence of tumor in the infratemporal fossa (fig. 6). There was no sign of tumor in the orbit, but the medial wall of the orbit seemed to be infiltrated. Linear tomography disclosed tumor infiltration of the bottom of the orbit but the bone defect in the posterior wall of the maxillary sinus was not clearly visible.

In the third case there was tumor involvement of the left maxillary sinus, the nasal cavity including the septum, the ethmoidal and the sphenoidal

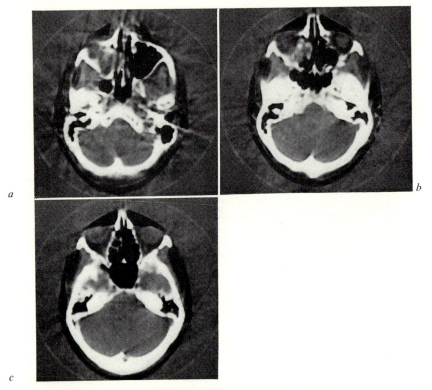

Fig.5. Maxillary carcinoma. *a* The left maxillary sinus is filled with tumor. Growth of tumor outside the sinus is well demonstrated. *b* There is some evidence of spread of the tumor to the bottom of the orbit. *c* There is no sign of involvement of the ethmoidal cells.

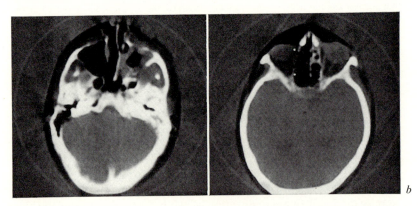

Fig.6. Maxillary carcinoma. *a* Postoperative bone defect in the anterior wall of the right maxillary sinus, and a wide opening medially, probably partly caused by the tumor. Bone destruction posteriorly with possible extension of the tumor to the infratemporal fossa. *b* There is no sign of tumor in the orbit, but the medial wall seems to be infiltrated.

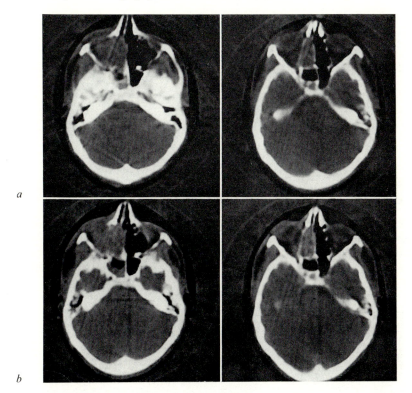

a

b

Fig. 7. Maxillary carcinoma. *a* There is tumor involvement of all the paranasal sinuses on the left side. *b* The attenuation was slightly increased after the injection of contrast medium.

cells (fig. 7). After the intravenous administration of 60 ml of Isopaque Cerebral (280 mg/ml) the visualization of the tumor tissue was slightly enhanced. Linear tomography gave no further information.

Fractures

Five cases with traumatic head injury and concomitant fractures of the facial bones are included in this study. In two cases there were comminuted fractures of the maxillae with varying degree of impaction of the anterior wall (fig. 8). Two cases showed extensive lesions of the nasal and the ethmoidal bones (fig. 9), and the remaining case had a depressed fracture of the frontal bone (fig. 10).

The transverse sections gave an exellent general view of the complex fractures of the facial bones including the sphenoid bone, and even minor

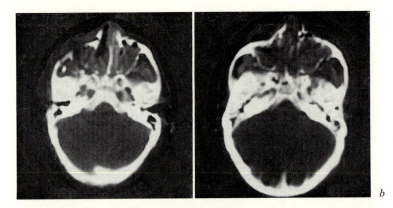

Fig.8. Two cases with comminuted fractures of the maxilla. *a* The anterior wall of the left maxillary sinus is impacted. Some air has escaped from the fractured sinuses into the swollen subcutaneous tissue. *b* The nasal cavity and the sinuses are almost completely filled with blood. There are also fractures of the right zygomatic arc with insignificant displacement.

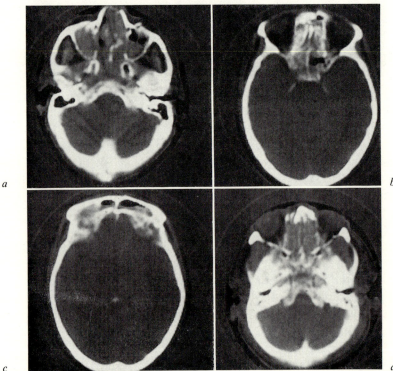

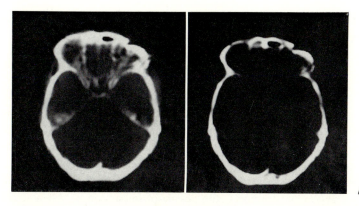

a   *b*

Fig. 10. Fractures of the frontal and the ethmoid bone. *a* The degree of depression may be satisfactorily assessed. *b* The same section displayed at another window level. The fragments appear more distinctly outlined.

fractures were well visualized. Displacement of the fragments, however, could not be fully evaluated without a supplementary plain film examination in the frontal projection.

Discussion

Carcinoma

In maxillary carcinoma an exact knowledge of the extent of the tumor, obtained by X-ray examination, forms a necessary basis for the designation of surgical and radiological treatment. With ordinary X-ray techniques, however, the spread of tumor outside the sinuses cannot be accurately defined. At computer tomography the attenuation values of the tumor did not appear to differ from that of the surrounding soft tissue. However, after the intravenous administration of a rather modest amount of contrast medium there was a slight increase of the attenuation values of the tumor tissue. Thus, contrast medium intravenously seems to enhance the visualization of a tumor, and the extent of tumor in the soft tissues may thereby be accurately settled. More-

---

Fig. 9. Two cases with fractures of the ethmoid and the nasal bones. *a* The displacement of the septum is clearly visible. *b* The uppermost part of the impacted nasal bones. Fracture of the right frontal sinus. *c* Fracture in the posterior wall of the left frontal sinus. Fluid in both frontal sinuses. Cerebrospinal rhinorrhoea was present in this case. *d* Another case with severe impaction of the nasal bones into the ethmoidal cells.

over, it may also be assumed that by the aid of contrast enhancement a malignant tumor could be differentiated from simple mucosal swelling, but this has not been investigated in the present study.

Fractures

Minute fractures of the thin bone plates of the paranasal sinuses, sometimes associated with cerebrospinal rhinorrhoea, quite often appear distinctly on computer tomography, while on plain films they may easily be overlooked. Similarly, very small volumes of intracranial air, often not clearly visible on plain films, may readily be identified on computer tomography.

In certain types of faciomaxillary fractures, for instance nasomaxillary and malar-zygomatic fractures, the degree of impaction is best assessed in axial projections, which closely correspond to the transverse sections in computer tomography. Plain film examination, as well as tomography, in axial projections is quite often impossible to carry out in seriously injured patients, and particularly in these cases computer tomography forms a convenient alternative method.

The method also entails considerable limitations, however. Thus, fractures running parallel to the sections are impossible to identify, unless significant displacement is present, and axial displacement, i.e. in a direction perpendicular to the sections, cannot be accurately assessed. This fact often makes a supplementary examination with conventional techniques necessary.

Summary

The diagnostic value of computer tomography in lesions of the paranasal sinuses has been investigated in three cases with maxillary carcinoma and in five cases with fractures of the facial bones. In most of the cases, particularly in carcinoma, computer tomography was found to provide additional information to that obtained with conventional X-ray techniques. In fractures, however, a supplementary plain film examination was found to be indispensable.

References

Liliequist, B. and Wickman, G.: A substitute for the waterbox in the original EMI brain scanner (to be published).

Dr. Å. Forssell, Department of Neuroradiology, University of Umeå, *S-901 85 Umeå* (Sweden)

Adv. Oto-Rhino-Laryng., vol. 24, pp. 51–57 (Karger, Basel 1978)

Congenital Deformity of the Internal Auditory Meatus and Labyrinth Associated with Cerebrospinal Fluid Fistula

PETER D. PHELPS and GLYN A. S. LLOYD

Department of Radiology, Royal National Throat, Nose and Ear Hospital, London

Introduction

Since removal of the fixed stapes became a common operation, it has been realised that there is a small percentage of patients undergoing stapedectomy in whom there is a profuse flow of perilymph or cerebrospinal fluid from the oval window. The mechanism of the 'stapes gusher' is uncertain but is believed to be due to an abnormal patency of the cochlear aqueduct [3]. Occasionally, a cerebrospinal fluid fistula may develop through the oval window spontaneously or as a result of minor head injury. These patients present with recurrent meningitis, cerebrospinal fluid rhinorrhoea or both. In every case there is congenital deformity of the inner ear on one side, but the congenital deafness is often overlooked or attributed to the meningitis and many fruitless investigations and operations are undertaken in an effort to find and stop the leak.

The path of the fistula in these congenital ear deformities from subarachnoid space to labyrinth through oval window to middle ear has been demonstrated in some cases by isotope or contrast cisternography [2, 11, 17, 18], or by direct observation at operation. In two cases [1, 7] a defect in the medial wall of the vestibule was observed through the oval window. Selective occlusion of the internal auditory meatus has been shown to stop the leak in some cases [4, 6], whilst in others blocking the cochlear aqueduct stopped the flow of cerebrospinal fluid [3]. However, few have had a full tomographic examination of the petrous temporal bones and consequently the descriptions of the inner ear deformity are vague.

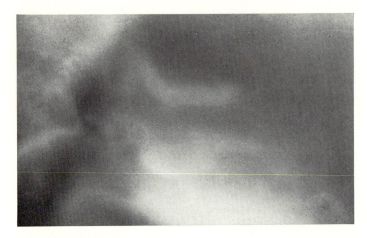

Fig.1. Dysplastic and dilated labyrinth with tapering internal auditory meatus.

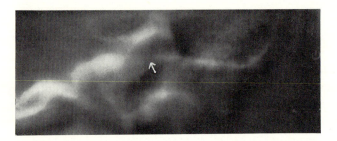

Fig.2. Another case with gross dilatation of the vestibule and lateral semicircular canal. The superior semicircular canal, however, appears normal. Note the large oval window (arrow).

Case Material

70 patients with congenital deformity of the bony labyrinth, internal auditory meatus, or both were reviewed. Seven patients were found to have a combination of inner ear deformities, repeatedly described as being associated with cerebrospinal fluid fistula. Two of these seven cases had in fact developed fistulae, one spontaneously and one as a result of surgical interference [6].

The most obvious feature was a general dilatation and dysplasia of the labyrinth (fig. 1). The vestibule was large with the lateral semicircular canal incompletely separated from it. The other semicircular canals were dilated in varying degree or appeared normal, (fig. 2). The cochlea lacked a modiolus and was in fact an amorphous sac of variable size, incompletely separated from the vestibule. The strangest feature, however, was the tapering internal auditory meatus, which was of normal width medially but narrowed towards its lateral end (fig. 3). In one case this type of inner ear deformity was bilateral.

Discussion

Many cochlear deformities are imprecisely described as being 'Mondini defects'. The type of cochlea shown in the original macroscopic dissection by MUNDINI and histological section by ALEXANDER consists of a basal turn and distal sac [16]. The internal auditory meatus is normal. JENSEN [8] has shown that the Mundini defect can be clearly demonstrated by tomography. As there is a relatively normal basal turn present some hearing is possible and indeed this has been shown in a few patients [12, 13, 15]. There is, however, a more severe type of deformity, for which JENSEN [9] suggests the term 'dysplasia', where the cochlea is represented by an amorphous sac which is often continuous with the dilated vestibule [1, 19]. This type of deformity is nearly always associated with a normal ear on the other side, so that the presence of complete unilateral deafness may not be appreciated. One case in our series had bilateral deformity and this appears to have been described once before [17]. A whole range of these cochlear deformities is present in anencephalics [20].

When a fistula develops through the oval or round window of a deformed labyrinth there is much argument as to whether the primary path from the subarachnoid space is via the cochlear aqueduct or the internal auditory meatus. There now seems little doubt that either or both routes may be involved.

FARRIOR and ENDICOTT [3] consider that most cases are due to dilatation of the cochlear aqueduct leading to perilymph hydrops and subsequent hearing loss. A deficient modiolus will of course mean that there is no helicotrema to restrict flow from the cochlear aqueduct to the oval window should a fistula develop. However, in most of the cases of spontaneous fistula described and always where the labyrinthine deformity is severe, the leak seems to be via the internal auditory meatus. GLASSCOCK [6] reviewed all known cases of fistulae with a deformed labyrinth and described a family, two of whom developed fistulae, in whom the lateral end of the internal auditory meatus was dilated.

CARTER et al. [2], who also reviewed all previously described cases, pro-

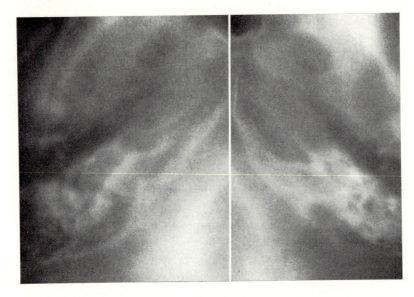

Base view

3a   Dysplastic   Normal

duced the only tomographic demonstration of contrast passing from the
internal auditory meatus to the labyrinth. This appeared to take place through
a defect in the lamina cribrosa in the region of the geniculate ganglion, but the
internal auditory meatus seemed to be narrowed at its lateral end as in our
patients. A few more cases have since been described which, from the tomograms used as illustrations, would seem to be further examples of this type of
lesion [1, 10, 14].

The subarachnoid space extends from the cerebellopontine angle for a
variable distance and may reach as far as the spiral and geniculate ganglia
(fig. 4). The modiolus or bony spiral not only forms the 'core' of the cochlea
but separates it from the internal auditory meatus. If the modiolus and spiral
ganglion are absent there will be a large defect in the lamina cribrosa through
which arachnoid can bulge and a fistula develop. The tapering of the lateral
end of the meatus tends to close this gap. If the cochlear sac is small and the

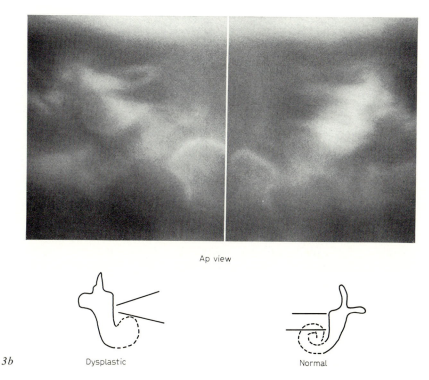

Ap view

3b   Dysplastic   Normal

Fig. 3. Frontal and base tomograms of a patient in whom the right cochlea is replaced by a large sac which is incompletely separated from the dilated vestibule and semicircular canals. The right internal auditory meatus narrows at its lateral end and communicates with the 'cochlea sac'. It also points somewhat posteriorly.

tapering marked closure may be complete, but if the sac is large and the 'compensatory' tapering inadequate then there would seem to be a risk of a fistula developing. A tapering internal auditory meatus probably occurs only with gross deformity of the cochlea. A funnel-sharped meatus is typically caused by an acoustic neuroma, but in such cases the appearance is due to widening of the medial end of the meatus, not narrowing of the lateral end.

Conclusion

We believe that there is a specific type of inner ear deformity charac-terised by: (1) a tapering internal auditory meatus, which narrows at its

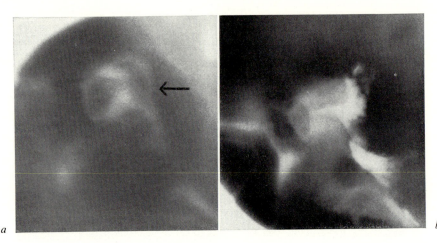

a   *b*

Fig.4. a An axial-pyramidal view of the cochlea sac, shown in figure 3. The internal auditory meatus (arrow) would appear to open into the sac, in the region of the geniculate ganglion. *b* Compare with the similar view of a normal inner ear. The extension of the sub-arachnoid space into the meatus is filled with Myodil and can be seen to extend as far as the spiral ganglion.

lateral end, and (2) generalised dilatation and dysplasia of the labyrinth. In particular the cochlea is an amorphous sac which completely lacks a modiolus. This is not the defect described by MUNDINI. Patients with this type of congenital inner ear malformation, which is probably more common than is generally realised, risk developing a cerebrospinal fluid fistula.

Summary

A type of inner ear deformity characterised by a tapering internal auditory meatus and dilated, dysplastic labyrinth was demonstrated by tomography in seven patients. Two of these developed cerebrospinal fluid fistulae through the oval window. The path of the fistula in this and other congenital deformities of the inner ear is discussed.

Acknowledgement

The illustrations were prepared by Miss M. P. OVERY, Department of Clinical Photography, The Institute of Laryngology and Otology, London.

References

1   BOTTEMA, T.: Spontaneous cerebrospinal fluid otorrhoea. Archs Otolar. *101:* 693–694 (1975).
2   CARTER, B.L.; WOLPERT, S.M., and KARMODY, C.S.: Recurrent meningitis associated with an anomaly of the inner ear. Neuroradiology *9:* 55–61 (1975).
3   FARRIOR, J.B. and ENDICOTT, J.N.: Congenital mixed deafness, cerebrospinal fluid otorrhea, ablation of the aqueduct of the cochlea. Laryngoscope *81:* 683–699 (1971).
4   FERRER, J.: Cerebrospinal otorrhea. Ann. Otol. Rhinol. Lar. *69:* 88–93 (1960).
5   FREELAND, A.P.: Non-traumatic CSF rhinorrhoea associated with congenitally malformed ears. J. Lar. Otol. *87:* 781–786 (1973).
6   GLASSCOCK, M.E.: The stapes gusher. Archs Otolar. *98:* 82–91 (1973).
7   GUNDERSEN, T. and HAYE, R.: Cerebrospinal otorrhea. Archs Otolar. *91:* 19–23 (1970).
8   JENSEN, J.: Malformations of the inner ear in deaf children. Acta radiol., suppl. *286,* pp. 11–90 (1969).
9   JENSEN, J.: Congenital anomalies of the inner ear. Radiol. Clin. N. Am. *12:* 473–482 (1974).
10 JONES, H.M. and CARR, R.: The problem of recurrent meningitis. Proc. R. Soc. Med. *67:* 1141–1143 (1974).
11 KAUFMANN, B.; JORDAN, V.M., and PRATT, L.L.: Positive contrast demonstration of a cerebrospinal fluid fistula through the fundus of the internal auditory meatus. Acta radiol. *9:* 83–90 (1969).
12 MUNDNICH, K.: The dysplasias of the middle and the inner ear in different types of malformation. Proc. R. Soc. Med. *67:* 1197–1199 (1974).
13 PAPARELLA, M.M. and ELFIKY, F.M.: Mondini's deafness. Archs Otolar. *95:* 134–140 (1972).
14 PARISIER, S.C. and BIRKIN, E.A.: Recurrent meningitis secondary to idiopathic oval window CSF leak. Laryngoscope *86:* 1503–1515 (1976).
15 PHELPS, P.D.; SHELDON, P.W.E., and LLOYD, G.A.S.: Hearing in patients with congenital deformity of the inner ear. Clin. Otolar. *1:* 31–38 (1976).
16 PHELPS, P.D. and WRIGHT, J.L.W.: Coils of the cochlea. Clin. Radiol. *27:* 415–419 (1976).
17 ROCKETT, F.X.; WITTENBORG, M.H.; SHILLITO, J., jr., and MATSON, D.D.: Panto-paque visualization of a congenital dural defect of the internal auditory meatus causing rhinorrhea. Amer. J. Roentg. *91:* 640–646 (1964).
18 STOOL, S.; LEEDS, N.E., and SULMAN, K.: The syndrome of congenital deafness and otic meningitis: diagnosis and management. J. Pediat. *71:* 547–552 (1967).
19 TSCHIANG, H.H.; SPENCER HARRISON, M., and OZSAHINAGLU, C.: Cerebro-spinal otorrhoea. J. Lar. Otol. *87:* 475–482 (1973).
20 WRIGHT, J.L.W.; PHELPS, P.D., and FRIEDMAN, I.: Temporal bone studies in anencephaly (1). J. Lar. Otol. *90:* 919–927 (1976).

Dr. P.D. PHELPS, Department of Radiology, Royal National Throat, Nose and Ear Hospital, *London* (England)

Adv. Oto-Rhino-Laryng., vol. 24, pp. 58–67 (Karger, Basel 1978)

Neurinomas of the Labyrinthine Portion of the Facial Nerve Canal

A Report of Two Cases

B. LILIEQUIST

Department of Diagnostic Neuroradiology (Director: B. LILIEQUIST),
University of Umeå, Umeå

Neurinomas arising from the seventh cranial nerve are rare and less than 100 cases are reported in the literature. Most facial neurinomas take their origin in the tympanic or mastoid portion of the facial nerve canal or peripherally. Those issuing from the first portion of the canal, the vicinity of the geniculate ganglion or from the great superficial petrosal nerve are rare. Facial neurinomas can also arise from the cisternal portion of the nerve or from its passage along the internal auditory canal.

Tumours arising from the tympanic and the vertical portion of the Fallopian canal usually grow into the middle ear, the mastoid cells or into the posterior fossa or they reach the region of the parotid gland. Neurinomas issuing from the geniculate ganglion, proximal to it or from the internal auditory canal either penetrate into the middle cranial fossa or are restricted to the canal. They seldom reach the posterior fossa in contrast to neurinomas arising from the cisternal part of the nerve which appears as a pontine angle tumour.

Very small tumours in the canal can be revealed only by the use of tomography of the various portions of the canal and their diagnosis is dependent upon a high degree of suspicion in the patient with a lower motor neuron facial paralysis as neoplastic involvement of the facial nerve is estimated to account for only 5% of all cases with facial palsy. On the other hand facial neurinomas can present themselves as an expanding lesion in the middle cerebral fossa.

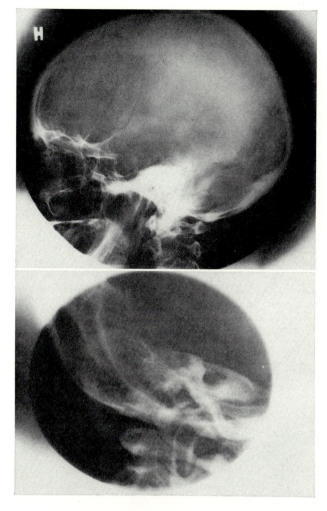

Fig. 1. Case 1. Plain skull examination. *a* Changes of sella turcica caused by increased intracranial pressure. *b* Destruction of anteromedial surface of the right temporal bone.

Case Reports

Case 1

42-year-old woman, who since 3 years had noted tinnitus and a progressive hearing loss on the right side. The last 9 months a facial palsy had appeared. On admission to the hospital there was a partial neurogenic hearing loss on the right side and a facial paresis. There was no stapedial reflex on either side and ice-water irrigation of the right ear showed

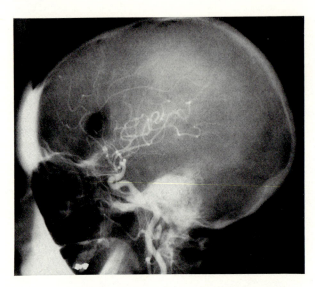

Fig. 2. Case 1. Carotid angiography. Avascular expanding lesion in the middle cranial fossa.

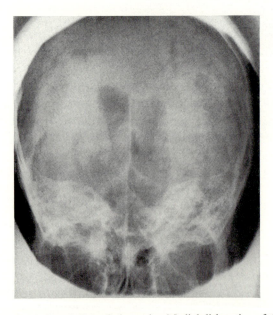

Fig. 3. Case 1. Encephalography. Medial dislocation of the right temporal horn.

no response. Examination of the intermedius nerve function showed an impaired lacrimal secretion on the right side. Test of chorda tympani function showed a complete loss of taste on the anterior two-thirds on the right half of the tongue. The chorda tympani function was also tested by examination of the submandibular secretion. Citric acid stimulation disclosed a very low secretion on the right side indicating total or subtotal disruption of the right chorda tympany secretory fibers. The left chorda tympani was normal as was also the reflectory parotid secretion bilaterally.

Roentgen examination of the skull and temporal bone showed changes in the sella turcica caused by raised intracranial pressure and a destruction of the anteromedial surface of the right temporal bone (fig. 1). Semicircular tomography showed that the destruction was located adjacent to the site of the geniculate ganglion and that it reached the inner auditory canal and the middle cranial fossa.

Carotid angiography performed on the right side showed an avascular expanding lesion in the middle cranial fossa (fig. 2). Encephalography did not disclose any change in the posterior cranial fossa but showed a dislocation of the right temporal horn medially and upwards (fig. 3).

There was no papilloedema and a lumbar puncture showed no rise in the amount of protein (36 mg%). The patient was subsequently operated upon through a right-sided subtemporal craniectomy. The tumour was found to be located extradurally in the middle fossa bulging from an eroded aperture in the temporal bone. It was seen to issue from the facial nerve just proximal to the geniculate ganglion and it also had an extension along the internal auditory canal reaching the meatus but not protruding through it. Histological examination verified the preoperative diagnosis of a neurinoma.

Case 2

A boy, 19 years of age, who since the age of 7 could not whistle, obviously due to a facial paresis. At the age of 16 he could no longer close his left eye. One year later a hearing loss on the left side was noted. The last year he suffered tinnitus and attacks of headache as well as tics. On admission to the hospital a lagophthalmos was noted on the left side as well as a peripheral left-sided facial palsy. There was an increased lacrimal secretion on the left side and a constant noise in the ear. There was no papilloedema. A partial upper homonymous hemianopsia to the right was also noted. Examination of the eighth nerve showed a hearing loss on the left side and a totally absent vestibular function. The stapedial reflex was lost in the left ear. Examination of the intermedius nerve function showed no secretion from the left submandibular gland and no taste on the anterior part of the tongue on the left side. The lacrimal secretion was diminished on the left side.

Roentgen examination of the skull and the temporal bone showed an extensive destruction of the left temporal bone including the tip of the petrous bone and the antero-medial portion of its bony walls as well as a large region of the floor of the middle fossa (fig. 4). The destruction reached the clivus medially and the cranial vault laterally. Technetium scintigraphy showed a tumour with extensive uptake of the isotope located to the middle cranial fossa (fig. 5).

Vertebral angiography showed a tumour in close vicinity to the tentorium but without any definite signs of a posterior fossa engagement (fig. 6). Carotid angiography showed a large expanding lesion in the middle fossa. The tumour was mainly avascular when examined from the internal carotid artery (fig. 7). Selective external carotid angiography disclosed a faint staining of the tumour and large veins on its surface (fig. 8).

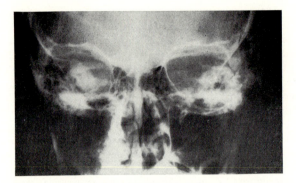

Fig. 4. Case 2. Destruction of the left temporal bone.

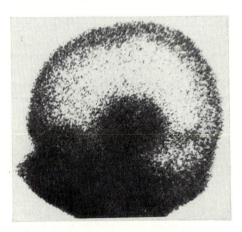

Fig. 5. Case 2. Technetium scintigram showing a tumour with extensive uptake of the isotope in the middle cranial fossa.

The preoperative diagnosis was a large facial neurinoma growing in the middle cranial fossa. A subtotal extirpation was performed of a huge extradurally located neurinoma, who reached the midline and the tentorial notch without penetrating into the posterior fossa. The tumour was adherent to the vault laterally and to the floor of the middle fossa and the temporal bone and a total extirpation was impossible. The tumour apparently issued from the facial nerve along its passage in the internal auditory canal. Histological examination confirmed the preoperative diagnosis of a neurinoma.

The cardinal signs and symptoms of a facial nerve tumour are facial palsy and a hearing loss, the leading one being dependent upon the site of the tumour along the facial nerve. Tumours issuing distal to the geniculate ganglion will not engage the great superficial petrosal nerve and therefore

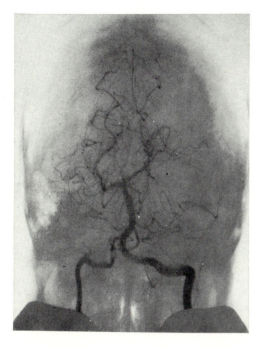

Fig.6. Case 2. Vertebral angiography. Avascular tumour in the vicinity of the tentorial notch.

the lacrimal secretion is not disturbed. Neurinomas arising from the intra-petrosal portion of the temporal bone in the vicinity of the geniculate ganglion can either penetrate into the middle fossa where they present with a distinct radiological and clinical picture or grow in the direction of the tip entirely inside the bone. In the literature so far 18 cases have been reported but cases with distinct expanding lesion in the middle fossa and a detailed report of the symptoms are restricted to 12 including the 2 cases reported here.

The clinical signs and symptoms of 12 facial neurinomas who had pro-truded into the middle cranial fossa are recorded in table I. A facial palsy was noted in all 12 cases with a duration between 9 months and 26 years. The facial paresis was of a progressive character in all patients with one exception where the paresis had a recurring course. All patients with excep-tion of 3 had a hearing loss with a duration between 1.5 and 15 years. Tinnitus was noted in 4 patients and pain was felt only in 1 patient. The vestibular

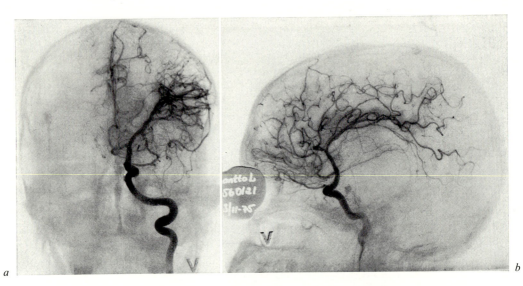

Fig. 7. Case 2. Internal carotid angiography. *a* A–P. *b* Lateral view. Large expanding avascular lesion in the middle cranial fossa.

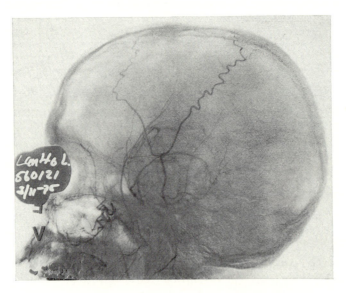

Fig. 8. Case 2. External carotid angiography. Faint staining of tumour with large veins on its surface.

Table I. Clinical signs recorded in 12 patients with facial neurinomas issuing from the labyrinthine portion of the facial canal

Clinical signs and symptoms	Pathologic	Normal	Not examined
7th nerve			
Facial palsy	12	–	–
Pain	1	11	
Tic	4	8	
Stapedial reflex	2		
8th nerve			
Hearing loss	9	12	
Tinnitus	4	8	
Inner ear	7	5	
N. petr. superf.			
Lacrimal secretion	6	2	4
Chorda tympani			
Anterior ageusia	9	1	2
Salivary secretion			
(submandibular and sublingual secretion)	5	1	6
Epileptic fits	3	9	
Choked discs	1	11	
Hemianopsia	2	10	
Spinal fluid examination	1	5	6

Table II. Result of roentgen examinations in 12 patients with facial neurinomas issuing from the labyrinthine portion of the facial canal

X-ray examination	Pathologic	Normal	Not examined
Skull ex. and/or tomography	7	4	1
Linear calcification middle fossa	3	8	1
Encephalography	2	–	10
Carotid a-y	6	–	6
Vertebral a-y	1	–	11
Scintography	2	–	10

function was lost in 8 patients. The taste was examined in 10 cases and found to be lost in 9. The salivary secretory function of the intermedius nerve was examined in 6 and affected in 5. The lacrimal secretion was examined in 8 and lost in 6. Epileptic fits was noted in 3 patients. The spinal fluid was examined in 7 patients and found to be normal in all except in 1 patient with a rise of the amount of protein (143 mg%). In 1 patient choked discs were noted and in 2 a hemianopsia was found.

Table II shows the result of X-ray examinations in the 12 cases. In 4 patients no changes were found. A curvilinear calcification could be seen in the middle cranial fossa in 3 patients. Encephalography is reported in 1 patient and showed a displacement of the temporal horn as did ventriculography in another patient. Cerebral angiography was employed in 6 patients and showed an expanding lesion in the middle cranial fossa in all cases. The isotope scintigraphy technique was used in 2 patients and was reported abnormal in both.

Conclusion

The combination of a facial palsy and a hearing loss with the presence of destructions in the anteromedial portion of the pyramid possibly with a linear calcification in the middle cranial fossa strongly favours a facial neurinoma.

The diagnostic procedure should include a complete hearing investigation, test of the vestibular and intermedius nerve function and a roentgenological examination including tomography of the temporal bone, possibly encephalography and angiography. In the future CT scan can probably replace angiography, and isotope scintigram as has been the case with acoustic nerve tumours as well as with tentorial meningiomas.

References

FURLOW, L.T.: The neurosurgical aspects of seventh nerve neurilemmoma. J. Neurosurg. *17:* 721 (1960).

HORA, J.F. and BROWN, A.K., jr.: Neurilemmoma of the facial nerve. Laryngoscope *74:* 134 (1964).

ISAMAT, F.: Neurinomas of the facial nerve. Acta neurochir. *31:* 268 (1975).

KLEINSASSER, O. und FRIEDEMANN, G.: Über Neurinoma des Nervus facialis. Zentbl. Neurochir. *19:* 49 (1959).

LILIEQUIST, B.; THULIN, C.-A.; TOVI, D.; WIBERG, A., and ÖHMAN, J.: Neurinoma of the labyrinthine portion of the facial nerve. Case report. J.Neurosurg. *37:* 105 (1972).
PULEC, J.L.: Facial nerve tumors. Ann.Otol.Rhinol.Lar. *78:* 962 (1969).
SCHNECK, S.A.; LAFF, H.I., and STEPEHNS, J.W.: Facial nerve tumors and progressive facial palsy. Archs Neurol. *2:* 452 (1960).
STEWART, B.M.: Recurrent facial palsy and tumor. Archs Otolar. *83:* 543 (1966).
TREMBLE, G.E. and PENFIELD, W.: Operative exposure of the facial canal with removal of a tumor of the greater superficial petrosal nerve. Archs Otolar. *23:* 573 (1936).

Dr. B. LILIEQUIST, Department of Diagnostic Neuroradiology, University of Umeå, *S-901 85 Umeå* (Sweden)

Adv. Oto-Rhino-Laryng., vol. 24, pp. 68–70 (Karger, Basel 1978)

Neuromas of the Facial Nerve

GALDINO E. VALVASSORI

Department of Radiology, University of Illinois, Chicago, Ill.

Intratemporal neuromas or neurilemmomas of the facial nerve are uncommon although not rare tumors. PULEC [1] in 1969 cited 74 cases from the literature and added another 11 cases. SAITO and BAXTER [3] found 5 small neuromas of the facial nerve as they reviewed 600 temporal bones at the Massachusetts Eye and Ear Infirmary, 4 which were completely asymptomatic.

It is the purpose of this presentation to report on 21 patients with intratemporal facial nerve neuromas diagnosed by the author during the past 10 years.

Clinical Findings

Neoplastic involvement of the facial nerve represents 5% of all lower motor neuron facial paralysis: of these, primary intratemporal tumors of the facial nerve comprise an even smaller number. The tumor is generally believed to arise from the sensory elements of the nerve. Three of our cases had a known history of neurofibromatosis with multiple neurofibromas in many peripheral nerves.

The clinical symptomatology depends upon the site of origin and the time of diagnosis of the lesion. It is obvious that the clinical findings are quite subtle whenever the lesion is small and still confined to the facial canal but becomes more severe and variable as the mass becomes larger and involves the adjacent structures.

In 11 cases, or more than half of the patients, the initial symptom was peripheral type of facial palsy, quite often of sudden onset and therefore simulating Bell's palsy. 1 patient developed a facial tic without paralysis. In 6 cases the clinical symptomatology simulated an acoustic neuroma. In 2 instances the only clinical finding was a conductive hearing loss produced by the encroaching of the mass upon the ossicular chain. Finally 1 patient had a palpable lump below the right ear lobe which had become progressively larger but had not caused a facial weakness.

The site of origin of the tumor in our series was as follows: (1) Limited to the fundus of the internal auditory canal only: 1 case. (2) Internal auditory canal and first or petrous segment of the facial canal: 5 cases. (3) Anterior genu (often involving the adjacent portion of the petrous and tympanic segments): 8 cases. (4) Tympanic segment: 4 cases. (5) Mastoid segment: 3 cases.

Radiographic findings

Conventional radiography is of limited value in the study of facial neuromas unless the mass has reached voluminous proportions. The only adequate way to properly study the facial canal is by multidirectional tomography. Sections 1 or 2 mm apart are obtained in the frontal and 20° coronal oblique projections for the study of the petrous and tympanic segments of the facial canal and lateral or modified lateral sections for the evaluation of the vertical or mastoid segment. Whenever the tumor arises or breaks into the internal auditory canal a posterior fossa myelogram is required to establish the size and extent of the intracanalicular mass. The radiographic findings range from a simple expansion of the facial canal to destruction of the adjacent portion of the petrous pyramid and mastoid as the tumor erodes through the canal wall. Whenever the tumor grows into the middle ear cavity a well-defined soft tissue mass is often recognizable. In 2 cases referred for pure conductive hearing loss without facial weakness we found a tumor arising from the tympanic segment of the nerve and eroding the long process of the incus.

Conclusion

Facial neuromas are uncommon but not rare tumors of the temporal bone. A tomographic study of the facial canal should be performed in all patients with facial paralysis, often diagnosed as Bell's palsy, presenting no improvement or recovery after 2 weeks and a progressive nerve degeneration as established by repeated electromyographic tests.

References

PULEC, J.L.: Facial nerve tumors. Transactions *57:* 167–187 (1969).

VALVASSORI, G.E.: Tumors involving the facial nerve canal. Excerpta Med.Int.Congr. Series No. *206*, p. 611 (1969).

SAITO, H. and BAXTER, A.: Undiagnosed intratemporal facial nerve neurilemmomas. Archs Otolar. *95:* 415–419 (1972).

NEELY, J.G. and ALFORD, B.R.: Facial nerve neuromas. Archs Otolar. *100:* 298–301 (1974).

Prof. G.E. VALVASSORI, Professor of Radiology, University of Illinois, *Chicago, Ill.* (USA)

Adv. Oto-Rhino-Laryng., vol. 24, pp. 71–93 (Karger, Basel 1978)

Tomography in Menière's Disease – Why and How

Morphological, Clinical and Radiographic Aspects

HERMANN F. WILBRAND, JAN STAHLE and HELGE RASK-ANDERSEN

Uppsala University Hospital, Uppsala

Introduction

Menière's disease in its characteristic triadic form presents typical vertiginous episodes, often associated with nausea and vomiting, tinnitus and progressive sensorineural hearing loss. Additional common symptoms are a sense of fullness in the ear and distortion of hearing, which may appear periodically. The most usual form of onset of the disease is simultaneous hearing loss and vertigo, which occurred in 41% of a large group of patients [ENANDER and STAHLE, 1967]. Vertigo alone was the initial symptom in 37%, while hearing loss alone was the least common of the first symptoms (22%).

In Sweden the disease is most often manifested in the fourth and fifth decades of life and it is equally common in both sexes [STAHLE, 1976]. The mean age on admission to hospital was 50 years in a large, selected series of severely disabled patients, all of whom were treated surgically [STAHLE, 1976]. In the British population the left inner ear has been reported to be more often involved [CAWTHORNE and HEWLETT, 1954], while in Sweden no such difference between the sides has been documented [STAHLE, 1976]. The frequency of involvement of both ears has been reported to be 25–43% [HARRISON and NAFTALIN, 1968; STAHLE, 1968; QUIST-HANSEN and HAYE, 1976; MORRISON, 1976] and increases with the duration of the illness [MORRISON, 1976; STAHLE, 1976].

The aetiology of the typical Menière's disease is unknown. A fairly good knowledge of the histopathology has been attained from the starting point of the classical and fundamental report of HALLPIKE and CAIRNS [1938]. The principal histological finding is a distension of the endolymphatic compartments, especially the cochlear duct and the saccule, due to an increase in the volume of endolymph (hydrops). Atrophy of the cochlear neurons of the apical turn, vestibular fibrosis and epithelial degeneration in the stria vascularis are other observations [SCHUKNECHT, 1974, 1976].

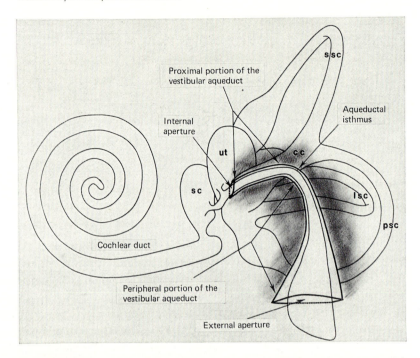

Fig. 1. The membranous labyrinth and the vestibular aqueduct. The aqueduct originates from the medial wall of the vestibule as a bony canal for the endolymphatic duct and
sac. The external aperture of the aqueduct is located on the posterior surface of the pyramid.
ssc = Superior semicircular canal, lsc = lateral semicircular canal, psc = posterior semicircular canal, cc = crus commune, ut = utriculus, sc = sacculus.

    The endolymphatic sac, which is a process of the membranous inner ear
and is located partly in the vestibular aqueduct and partly between two dural
sheets on the posterior surface of the pyramid, is thought to play a fundamental
role in inner ear metabolism and is believed to be involved in the pathogenesis
of Menière's disease. The variational anatomy of the vestibular aqueduct
with the endolymphatic duct and sac has been described in earlier papers
[STAHLE and WILBRAND, 1974a, b; WILBRAND *et al.*, 1974].

    The endolymphatic sac is connected with the rest of the inner ear by the
endolymphatic duct, originating from the saccule and utricle (fig. 1). Endolymph secreted in the stria vascularis is believed to flow through the endolymphatic duct to the endolymphatic sac. In the richly plicated epithelial
lined proximal part of the sac, the *pars rugosa,* absorption of endolymph and
phagocytosis of debris are supposed to take place.

Table I. Visibility of the vestibular aqueduct on tomograms, expressed as the percentage number of ears with visible aqueducts

Healthy subjects	Patients with Menière's disease (86 ears)		
(32 ears)	unilaterally diseased		bilaterally
	non-diseased ear	diseased ear	diseased
100%	65%	59%	53%

Disturbances in this 'longitudinal endolymph flow', due to obstruction of the endolymphatic duct or deficient absorption of endolymph in the sac, may contribute to the development of Menière's disease. Such disturbances may be caused by perisaccular fibrosis resulting in impairment of the blood supply of the endolymphatic duct and sac [HALLPIKE and CAIRNS, 1938; WITTMAACK, 1956; ALTMANN and ZECHNER, 1968; SHAMBAUGH et al., 1969], or in rare cases by bony obstruction [CLEMIS and VALVASSORI, 1968; GUSSEN, 1971].

The vestibular aqueduct, which is the bony canal housing the endolymphatic duct and part of the sac, has been studied intensively by various techniques during the last decade in an attempt to get better insight into the pathogenesis of Menière's disease [ANSON, 1965; ZECHNER and ALTMANN, 1969]. The first tomographic reproductions and descriptions of the vestibular aqueduct were presented by CLEMIS and VALVASSORI [1968], who suggested that there was a correlation between an invisible aqueduct and this disease. This observation has been verified in several later reports [BRÜNNER and PEDERSEN, 1971; VALVASSORI, 1974; RUMBAUGH et al., 1974; ØIGAARD et al., 1975]. Although there is a high frequency of radiographically non-visible aqueducts, this feature is not pathognomonic for Menière's disease, but has also been reported in chronic middle ear diseases [ØIGAARD et al., 1975]. In contrast to the tomographic observations, YUEN and SCHUKNECHT [1972] have found normally patent aqueducts at histology in 19 Menière ears.

Our previous findings concerning the visibility of the vestibular aqueduct on tomograms are summarized in table I. It was visible in all healthy individuals, while in patients with Menière's disease it could be seen in only 59% on the diseased side.

Studies of the vestibular aqueduct by means of plastic moulding of the inner ear, microdissection of human temporal bone specimens and tomography of temporal bone specimens as well as of healthy individuals have formed a basis for our assessment of the temporal bone pathology in patients with Menière's disease [STAHLE and WILBRAND, 1974 a, b; WILBRAND et al., 1974; RASK-ANDERSEN et al., 1977; WILBRAND, 1977].

This paper will present (1) our common aims with respect to inner ear tomography and some results of previous investigations and (2) a description of the tomographic procedure. We studied the temporal bones in Menière's disease by tomography in order to gain (1) fundamental knowledge of the appearances of the temporal bone in Menière's disease, and subsequently to find out (2) what roentgen-anatomic structures evaluable by tomography will be of interest in otosurgery for Menière's disease.

Morphological Aspects

Previous investigations on patients with Menière's disease have indicated certain pathological characteristics that may be revealed by tomography and verified at operation. These observations initiated a study on temporal bone specimens with emphasis upon the variational anatomy of the vestibular aqueduct and its surrounding structures [RASK-ANDERSEN et al., 1977]. 48 human temporal bone specimens were tomographed and subsequently dissected by means of a dental drill, using osmic acid for tracing the contents of the vestibular and cochlear aqueducts and their respective accessory canals. Topographic studies of the inner ear lumina were also carried out on 12 plastic moulds of tomographed human temporal bones [WILBRAND, 1977].

The general anatomical appearance of the vestibular aqueduct is that of a bony canal arising from the medial wall of the vestibule, running fairly parallel to the crus commune through the otic capsule to a bend, whence it changes its course downward and more laterally to the external aperture on the posterior face of the pyramid. The angle between the proximal and peripheral portions is about 90° (fig. 1–3). The gradual flat widening of the

---

Fig. 2. Type 1 – large cell periaqueductal pneumatization, left ear. *a* Posterior view showing the course of the vestibular aqueduct (VA) as it passes under the posterior semi-circular canal (PSCC) towards the common crus and enters the vestibule. The external aperture (EA) is wide (7 mm). The extent and position of the large round foveate impression is indicated with arrows. Incidentally, the transverse crest (TC) and so-called Bill's bar (BB) within the internal acoustic meatus (IAM) are excellently reproduced. *b* Surgeon's view of the same bone, showing the size and positional relationship to the semicircular canals of EA and foveate impression (FI) as outlined, projected from the posterior view. Note how close FI lies to an imaginary line extended from the lateral semicircular canal (LSCC). JB = Region of the jugular bulb.

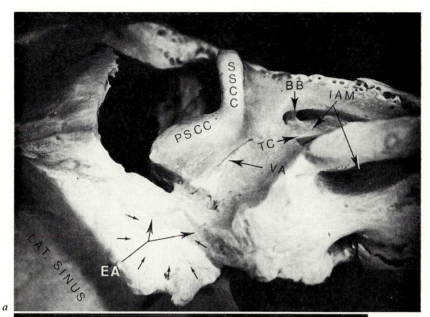

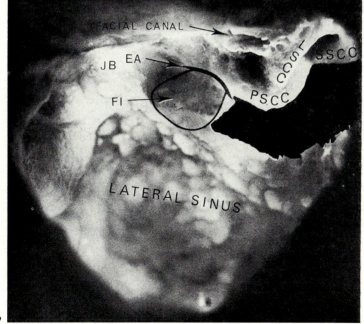

peripheral portion of the aqueduct houses part of the endolymphatic sac. The extraosseous part of the endolymphatic sac is located in a more or less pronounced foveate impression beneath the external aperture (fig. 2, 3). In pyramids with well developed peri- and infralabyrinthine pneumatization, the peripheral portion of the aqueduct has a long and flat spacious lumen (fig. 9). In poorly pneumatized pyramids with sparse or no periaqueductal air cells, the peripheral portion of the aqueduct is shorter, the triangular widening less spacious and the external aperture correspondingly smaller (fig. 10). In a few cases, however, the peripheral portion may show a recess-like widening located close to the posterior semicircular canal.

Another variety – often met in cases of Menière's disease – is a vestibular aqueduct with a narrow, short peripheral portion combined with a total lack of periaqueductal pneumatization. In these cases the peripheral portion often follows a curvilinear course through the pyramid, close to the posterior semicircular canal. The external aperture is then small and located high up on a steep posterior slope of the pyramid. The operculum will be represented by a thin bone lamella (fig. 10). This type of aqueduct can be found together with a fairly highly located jugular fossa (fig. 4), in the direct neighbourhood of the labyrinth and middle ear space. Between these two extremes (the very long aqueduct in a well-pneumatized pyramid and the very short one in a pyramid with a total lack of pneumatization medial to the arcuate eminence) the aqueductal length and shape vary according to the degree of peri- and infralabyrinthine pneumatization and to the size and location of the jugular fossa (fig. 9, 10).

Besides these normal variations, another type of aqueduct may be encountered (in fairly well pneumatized temporal bones), with a very narrow lumen of its peripheral portion but a fully developed length. Such an aqueduct offers only a narrow pathway for the endolymphatic duct and it seems unlikely that any space will be lent to an endolymphatic sac.

Fig. 3. Type 3 – absence of periaqueductal air cells, left ear. *a* Posterior view showing the shorter vestibular aqueduct (VA) and the high, narrow external aperture (EA; 2.5 mm) with a shallow, elongated foveate impression (arrows). Note that this type 3 specimen had to be rotated slightly to best visualize the most direct course of the vestibular aqueduct. *b* Surgeon's view of the same bone, showing the pronounced inferiorly positioned foveate impression (FI) and the very narrow EA projected from the posterior view and outlined. The FI and presumably the endolymphatic sac are elongated and project towards the region of the jugular bulb (JB). It lies inferior to an imaginary line extended from the lateral semicircular canal (LSCC). This type is characteristic for patients with long-standing Menière's disease.

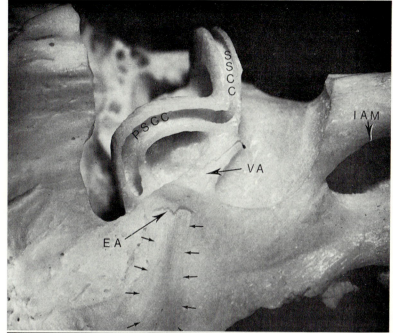

a

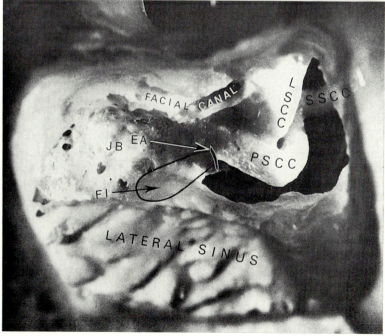

b

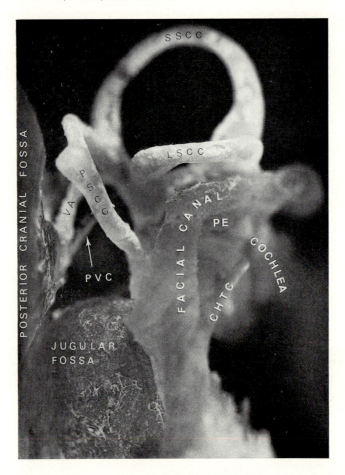

Fig. 4. Plastic mould of a human right inner ear. With type 3 periaqueductal pneumatization the jugular fossa may be located extremely high up in the temporal bone, close to the vestibular aqueduct and the posterior semicircular canal. The distance between the PSCC and the posterior cranial fossa is very short, which means a narrow operation field. PVC–paravestibular canaliculus, VA = vestibular aqueduct, PSCC = posterior semicircular canal, CHTC = chorda tympani canal, PE = pyramidal eminence.

A paravestibular or accessory canaliculus arises from the medial wall of the vestibule in the close vicinity of the proximal portion of the vestibular aqueduct (fig. 4–6, 9, 10). The canaliculus runs more or less in parallel to the aqueduct. It opens directly in or near the foveate impression below the external aperture of the aqueduct.

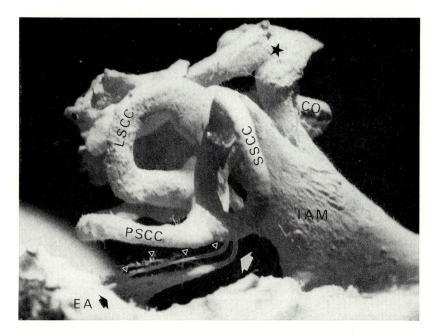

Fig. 5. Plastic mould of the human left inner ear with type 1 periaqueductal pneumatization seen from above. The vestibular aqueduct (large white arrow) has a right-angle bend between its proximal and peripheral portions. It shows a gradual widening of its peripheral portion, with a straight course, and opens at the posterior surface of the pyramid in the external aperture (EA). The large white arrow points at the bend of the vestibular aqueduct. The adjacent paravestibular canaliculus, which runs close to the posterior semicircular canal (PSCC) is indicated by four white triangles. Its distal portions is split into two branches. IAM = Internal acoustic meatus, CO = cochlea. The upper facial knee is marked with an asterisk.

Tomographic Information

At tomography variations in the peri- and infralabyrinthine pneumatization of the temporal bone are easily distinguished (fig. 7, 8). In healthy individuals this pneumatization exhibits some relation to the extent of the mastoid cell formation. Three different types of periaqueductal pneumatization have been identified in our investigations: type 1, with large-cell pneumatization; type 2, with small air cells or bone marrow spaces (which cannot be differentiated from each other by tomography); and type 3, showing a complete absence of air cells [STAHLE and WILBRAND, 1974 a, b]. These different types of peri- and infralabyrinthine air cell formation, together with varying sizes

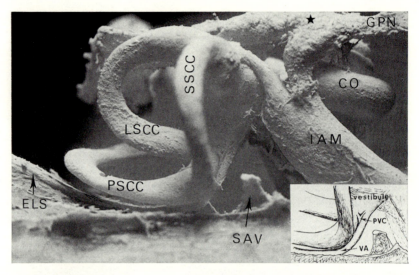

Fig. 6. Plastic mould of the human left inner ear with type 3 periaqueductal pneumatization, seen from above. The vestibular aqueduct (VA) runs from the vestibule with a curved course to the external aperture on the posterior surface of the pyramid. The peripheral part has a curvilinear course. The endolymphatic sac (ELS) is partly located in the peripheral, wider part of the vestibular aqueduct. The aqueduct is accompanied by the paravestibular canaliculus or accessory canal (PVC), which originates with two branches from the medial wall of the vestibule (see insert). PSCC = posterior semicircular canal, IAM = internal acoustic meatus, CO = cochlea, GPN = canal for the greater petrosal nerve, SAV = canal for the subarcuate vessels, * = 'upper knee' of the facial canal.

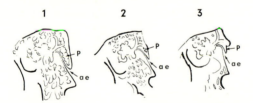

Fig. 7. Different types of periaqueductal pneumatization: (1) large cell pneumatization in the vicinity of the aqueduct, (2) small cell pneumatization in the vicinity of the aqueduct, (3) absence of air cells. P = Pneumatization, ae = external aperture of the vestibular aqueduct.

and positions of the jugular fossa, seem to have an influence both upon the appearance and shape of the vestibular aqueduct and upon its course through the pyramid. The vestibular aqueduct is longer and its external aperture wider in a type 1 pyramid and exhibits a tomographically readily identified bend of about 90° between its proximal and peripheral portions. In a type 3 pyramid,

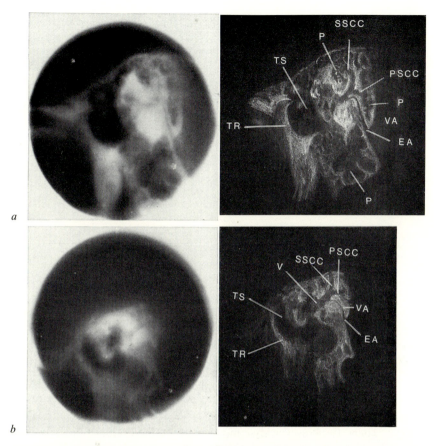

Fig.8a,b. Type 1 and type 3 periaqueductal pneumatization. Tomograms and corresponding drawings for orientation demonstrate the tomographic characteristics as well as the differences in pattern of the periaqueductal pneumatization. They show the size and presence of air cells, and the appearance and course of the vestibular aqueduct (VA) as well as the external aperture (EA). The longest VA is seen in type 1. In type 3 the VA is not only shorter but it is also curvilinear, with no definite straight distal portion. TS = tympanic space, V = vestibule, SSCC = superior semicircular canal, PSCC = posterior semicircular canal, TR = tympanic ring, P = pneumatic cells.

the aqueduct is shorter; it also shows a narrow external aperture and both its proximal and peripheral portions are curved without any clearly identifiable angulation between them. Frequently also the peripheral portion of the aqueduct shows a curvilinear course through the pyramid.

The type 1 pneumatization, which is common in healthy individuals

Table II. Tomographic classification of the type of periaqueductal pneumatization of the petrous pyramid and the length of the vestibular aqueduct in a normal population compared with patients with Menière's disease

	Type 1 large cell pneumatization	Type 2 small cell pneumatization	Type 3 no pneumatization
Normal subjects (n = 32 ears)	11	14	7
Length of the vestibular aqueduct, mm	10.3	8.2	7.4
Range, mm	7.2–13.5	6.1–9.9	6.7–8.1
Percent	34	44	22
Menière's disease (n = 86 ears)	0	28	58
Length of the vestibular aqueduct, mm	0	7.7	6.9
Range, mm		5.9–11.7	4.3–10.2
Percent	0	26	74

(table II), has been found in only a few patients with Menière's disease, in an early phase. Whether differences in the morphology of the pyramids between healthy individuals and patients with long-standing Menière's disease are due to a congenital factor or to a dynamic process of bone remodelling is unknown. There are, however, dynamic changes in the extent of bone marrow spaces in the pyramid. Whether once established pneumatization may decrease is not reported.

The extraosseous part of the endolymphatic sac is located in a foveate impression, which is represented by a shallow deepening in the posterior bony plate of the pyramid inferior to the external aperture of the vestibular aqueduct. Tomographic reproduction of the external aperture facilitates appraisal of the foveate impression, which varies in shape and appearance according to the different types of peri- and infralabyrinthine pneumatization. The type 1 pyramid has a wide and rounded foveate impression; in a type 3 pyramid it may appear as an elongated and narrow concavity inferior to the narrow external aperture (fig. 2, 3).

The three types are easily identified in tomograms, since the well-pneumatized large cell type (type 1) displays a well-developed air cell distribution in the operculum, whereas in type 3 the operculum is represented either by a

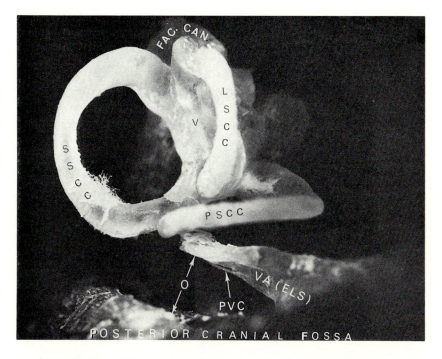

Fig.9. Plastic mould of a human right inner ear in the surgeon's transmastoid view. This is an example of type 1 periaqueductal pneumatization. The opercular volume (0) is quite large, with a marked distance between the vestibular aqueduct (VA(ELS)) and the posterior cranial fossa. The peripheral portion of the vestibular aqueduct is more voluminous in type 1. PVC = Paravestibular canal, V = vestibule, PSCC = posterior semicircular canal, LSCC = lateral semicircular canal, SSCC = superior semicircular canal, FAC. CAN. = facial canal.

very short and concrete bony plate or by a bony plate which is very thin but somewhat longer (fig. 7, 9, 10).

In type 1 and type 2 pyramids the course of the vestibular aqueduct can readily be discerned (both its proximal and peripheral portions) in one single tomogram, provided a suitable projection is chosen [CLEMIS *et al.*, 1968; BRÜNNER, 1971; WILBRAND *et al.*, 1974]. Easy reproduction is obtained when the aqueduct through the pyramid has a straight course (fig. 5, 8). Because of the small dimensions of the proximal portion of the aqueduct and of the bend between its proximal and peripheral portions [ANSON, 1968; CLEMIS and VALVASSORI, 1968; WILBRAND *et al.*, 1974], these structures need to be placed in the tomographic plane in order to be demonstrated. This is guaranteed by the choice of a 0.5-mm distance between the tomographic cuts. With a longer distance the aqueduct may not be reproduced in its entire length and difficulties may be encountered in visual perception of parts of this structure. The short distance between the cuts also allows metric estimation of the width of the external aperture from a series of cuts, which will be of value to the surgeon. Also valuable is knowledge of the location of the external aperture in relation to the posterior semicircular canal, together with metric information on the aqueductal length. In type 3 temporal bones the course of the peripheral portion of the aqueduct through the pyramid may be curvilinear (fig. 6). Such digression from a straight course creates difficulties in exact tomographic positioning. This is usually the reason for failure to reproduce the aqueduct and probably explains the high frequency of non-visible aqueducts reported in cases of Menière's disease [RUMBAUGH et al., 1974, STAHLE and WILBRAND, 1974 a, b; VALVASSORI, 1974]. High density of the petrous bone may also be responsible for non-visualization of the aqueduct.

Taking into consideration the above factors and using an optimum technique, we have recently been able to reproduce the aqueduct in its entire course in 65% in the diseased ears and in 80% in the non-diseased ears. These may be compared with our previous figures of 59 and 65%, respectively.

Clinical Aspects

Tomographic Findings Related to Inner Ear Function
Our intention has been to study the inner ear function in patients with Menière's disease on the basis of the tomographic visibility of the vestibular aqueduct. CLEMIS and VALVASSORI [1968] have reported a high correlation between abnormal hearing and a non-visible aqueduct. We have compared

Fig. 10. Plastic moulds. a The right ear seen from above, this is an example of type 3 periaqueductal pneumatization. The opercular volume (0) is small with a very little distance between the peripheral portion of the vestibular aqueduct (VA) and the posterior cranial fossa. The vestibular aqueduct is accompanied by its paravestibular canal (PVC). The origin of the aqueduct from the medial wall of the vestibule (V) is readily seen as well as the course of the aqueducts proximal portion nearly parallel to the crus commune of the posterior (PSCC) and superior (SSCC) semicircular canals. LSCC = Lateral semicircular canal, IAM = internal acoustic meatus. b The same right ear from the surgeons transmastoid view. The opercular volume (0) is quite small in the type 3 periaqueductal pneumatization and consistent with the absence of periaqueductal air cells. The proximity of the vestibular aqueduct (VA) to the jugular fossa is apparent. The peripheral portion of the vestibular aqueduct houses part of the endolymphatic sac (ELS).

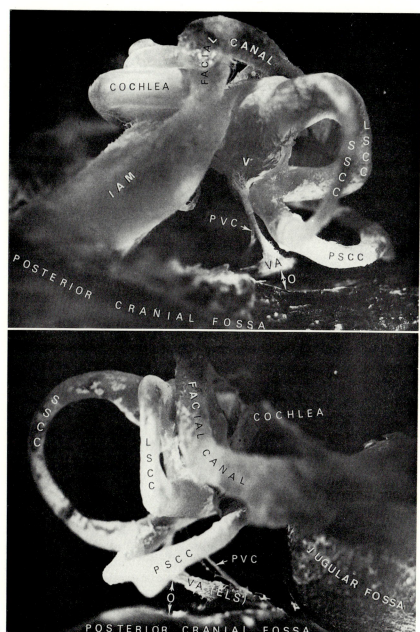

Table III. Visible/non-visible vestibular aqueducts in Menière's disease compared with age, duration and inner ear function

Age of patient	no correlation
Hearing loss	no correlation
Caloric response	no correlation
Duration of disease	pos. correlation (p = 0.05)

hearing (pure tone audiogram and discrimination score) and caloric response with the radiographic results, without finding any obvious relationships (table III). This means that severe hearing loss is not necessarily accompanied by a non-visible vestibular aqueduct. Neither was any correlation found between the tomographic visibility of the aqueduct and the age of the patient; thus a high age was not reflected by a non-visible vestibular aqueduct. On the other hand, the visibility is definitely influenced by the duration of the disease – the more long-standing the disease, the higher the frequency of patients with tomographically non-visible vestibular aqueducts. This may indicate a slow, progressive remodelling of the pyramid during the illness.

Endolymphatic Sac Surgery

Among several surgical methods for Menière's disease, surgery of the endolymphatic sac has seen a resurgence during the last few years as being a method not only producing relief from vertigo but also improving hearing loss in properly selected patients [ARENBERG *et al.*, 1977a; MORRISON, 1976]. Whatever method of sac surgery is used, preoperative information on some key landmarks, provided by tomography, is of great help to the surgeon. The anatomical structures of interest are the semicircular canals, the vestibular aqueduct and its external aperture, the cochlea, the facial canal, the lateral sinus and the jugular fossa (fig. 2–4). Short distances between the posterior semicircular canal and the posterior bony plate of the pyramid, and between the external aperture of the vestibular aqueduct and the jugular fossa, mean a narrow operation field (fig. 3, 4, 6, 10).

After having exposed the posterior fossa dura completely through the mastoid, the endolymphatic sac can be readily identified as a thick, whitish triangular or fan-shaped structure lying obliquely inferior in patients with Menière's disease. There is a thin, translucent, bluish dura mater on either side of the sac. The bluish dura mater can be readily depressed at all points, except where the endolymphatic sac and its vessels enter the temporal bone (fig. 12a). Often a bony ledge can be palpated beneath the sac. This is the external

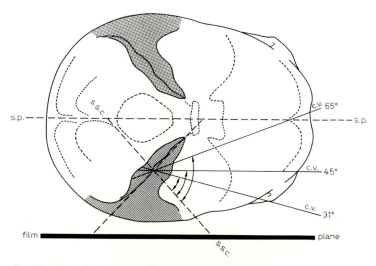

Fig. 11. Orientation of the vestibular aqueduct in reference to the superior semicircular canal in the skull base. The mean inclination of the vestibular aqueduct (C. V.) is 45° (range 31–65°) in reference to the plane of the superior semicircular canal (s.s.c.). On the assumption that the superior semicircular canal is located perpendicularly to the longitudinal axis of the pyramid, at an inclination of 45° to the sagittal plane of the skull base, the course of the vestibular aqueduct is, on the average, parallel to the film plane in the true lateral projection.

opening of the aqueduct. Once the sac is identified and completely exposed ('decompressed'), sac surgery can proceed. In Uppsala we have experience of two different methods of drainage operations [ARENBERG *et al.*, 1977b] which consist in the insertion of a silastic implant through an incision in the lateral sac wall into the lumen (fig. 12b). One of the implants is a so-called uni-directional inner ear valve, which is marked with radiopaque substance. This allows a postoperative check of the location of the implant (fig. 13). The other implant is a thin silastic strip with its tail ending in the mastoid cavity.

Remarks on the Tomographic Technique for
Reproducing the Vestibular Aqueduct

The tomographic technique is based on either hypocycloid or spiral movement of the tomographic system and the use of a 0.3-mm focal spot. A compatible photographic system is of major importance. Satisfactory craniostasis is often still a problem. The 'complete mechanics' of the tomographic system should be checked from time to time. This may be done either by the Funck test or by other means. The most sensible test in our opinion is to check the homogeneity and stability of the tomographic plane by means of a test object containing metal balls arranged in one plane in an arithmetic order. Such a device also allows an estimation of the 'layer thickness' when placed at an angle of 2–4° to the tomographic plane. Using a simple formula the layer thickness of the metal balls can be estimated [WILBRAND, 1975].

The head is placed either in the true lateral or in a modification of the lateral position (fig. 11) [WILBRAND *et al.*, 1974; STAHLE and WILBRAND, 1974a, b]. When in an examination of a temporal bone the tomographic plane approaches the assumed location of the vestibular aqueduct as it arises from the vestibule along with the *crus commune,* a 0.5-mm distance between the cuts must be chosen; otherwise the proximal portion and even part of the peripheral portion might not be visualized. The same is valid for tomography of similar minor details such as the stapes. Such objects are reproduced only when they lie in the tomographic plane to their fullest possible extent. Thus appropriate positioning is mandatory for successful reproduction of the aqueduct. This is best guaranteed when the aqueduct in its entire length is reproduced in one single tomogram (fig. 8). Since this is not always feasible, because of a sometimes curvilinear course of the aqueducts peripheral portion (fig. 6), not only the 0.5-mm distance between the cuts, but also optimum viewing conditions are necessary. Thus the tomograms should be viewed with their direct environment shaded with 1.5–1.8 densities at an ordinary viewing box.

Comments

Tomography in cases of Menière's disease has proved to be a valuable source of information in basic research. Comparative tomographic investigations of healthy subjects and patients with this disease have revealed marked differences in the gross anatomy of the pyramid, concerning its pneumatization and the corresponding appearance and shape of the vestibular aqueduct and its topographic relation to the surrounding inner ear structures. There has

---

Fig. 12. Saccotomy. *a* The endolymphatic sac has been exposed through an extended mastoidectomy in a patient with Menière's disease with type 3 periaqueductal pneumatization. The posterior fossa dura has been completely exposed. The bluish, thin dura mater (asterisks) can be readily depressed at all points except where the endolymphatic sac and its vessels enter the temporal bone through the external aperture of the vestibular aqueduct

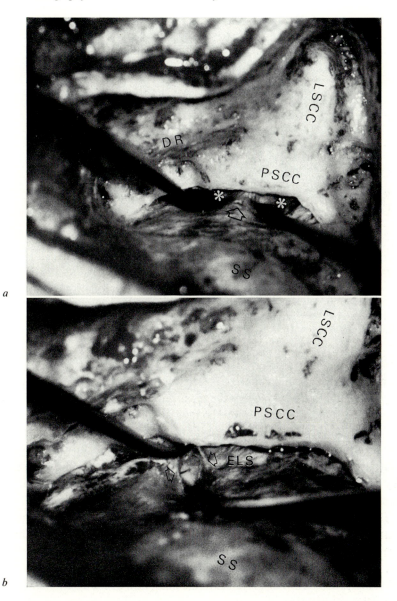

(arrow). SS = Sigmoid sinus, DR = digastric ridge, PSCC = posterior semicircular canal, LSCC = lateral semicircular canal. *b* In the next step of the same operation the lateral wall of the endolymphatic sac (ELS) has been incised, demonstrating a patent lumen (between the two arrows). In patients with Menière's disease the endolymphatic sac lies more inferiorly than in normal individuals.

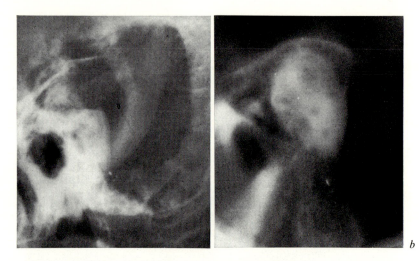

a   *b*

Fig. 13. Postoperative radiographic check of the position of the radioopaque sac implant. *a* Lateral view, plain radiography, showing a large operation cavity and a prominent otic capsule. On the lower posterior surface of the pyramid the implant is seen oriented towards the external aperture. *b* A tomogram at the level of the implant shows the implant to be in a correct position beneath the external aperture of the vestibular aqueduct.

been a widespread opinion that non-visibility of the vestibular aqueduct in tomograms might be of value as a diagnostic aid, but this view has not been corroborated. Non-visibility cannot be interpreted directly as bony changes in the vestibular aqueduct. Such a concept is still not confirmed, either by surgery or histology. Failure to reproduce the vestibular aqueduct tomographically can primarily be explained by faults in the tomographic technique or by unusual anatomic features (table IV). In only a few cases can it be expected that this failure is due to bony changes in the aqueduct.

Tomography of the vestibular aqueduct is also of diagnostic value in cases of sensorineural hearing loss [PHELPS, 1976; VALVASSORI, 1976], showing malformation and widening of the aqueductal lumina and other inner ear structures. The authors have encountered two cases of inexplicable sensorineural hearing loss, which both displayed extreme dilatation of the vestibular aqueduct on the affected side.

It has been stated that a tomographically non-reproduced vestibular aqueduct combined with low-grade pneumatization is not specific of Menière's disease, since corresponding tomographic findings may also be made in cases of chronic middle ear disease [ØIGAARD *et al.*, 1975]. It must be pointed out,

Table IV. Technical and anatomical factors reducing tomographic reproducibility of the vestibular aqueduct

Technical factors	Anatomical factors
1 'Incomplete mechanics', i.e. mechanical or geometrical failure in the tomographic system	Variations of inclination of the long axis of the pyramid to the sagittal plane of the skull, influencing positioning
2 Too large focal size of the roentgen tube	A short aqueduct having a peripheral portion with a curvilinear course
3 Too large distance between the tomographic cuts	The 'narrow lumen aqueduct'
4 Unfavourable positioning of patient	Extremely high density of petrous bone

however, that *the non-diseased ear in Menière's disease also often has a characteristic radiographic appearance similar to that of the diseased ear.* This abnormality in a clinically still healthy inner ear might be predictive of future clinical symptoms. Tomography is therefore also of value as a screening method.

Another observation is also frequently made in Menière's disease, namely a fairly well developed mastoid pneumatization but a sparse or complete lack of peri- and infralabyrinthine air cell formation. In such cases the course of the vestibular aqueduct through the pyramid renders reproduction of the aqueduct difficult. It is therefore stressed that for reproduction of the aqueduct in its entire length it needs to be placed to its fullest possible extent in the tomographic plane. A distance of 0.5 mm between the cuts is obligatory if reproduction of both the proximal and peripheral portion in one single tomogram is to be achieved. The proximal portion and the bend of the aqueduct are to date still near the borderline of tomographic reproducibility, because of their dimensions. More attention should also be paid to the principles of visual perception in radiography [TUDDENHAM, 1957; RÖHLER, 1967].

An observation not only of clinical interest but also of value in basic research is that patients with Menière's disease often had a shorter vestibular aqueduct on tomograms than healthy subjects (table II) and that patients with long-standing Menière's disease had a shorter vestibular aqueduct and a tendency towards non-visualization of the aqueduct compared with patients with only a short history. The duration of the disease was 6.7 years for visualized vestibular aqueducts, as compared with 10.7 years for non-visualized aqueducts.

Preoperative tomography in combination with basic studies on temporal bone specimens has already contributed valuable information about variations

in the location of the endolymphatic sac and the external aperture of the vestibular aqueduct. This information has facilitated identification of the endolymphatic sac in drainage operations. In Menière's disease the endolymphatic
sac and the vestibular aqueduct have a slightly modified size, location and
course as compared with normal individuals. Thus, in the surgeons view the
sac is more inferiorly positioned than in normal persons. This information has
been put to use in 49 consecutive operations on the endolymphatic sac, which
has been identified in all cases. This contrasts with reports in the literature
that the sac was absent, rudimentary, atrophic, agenic or impossible to
delineate at surgery in 5–30% [ARENBERG et al., 1977]. It is also our opinion
that preoperative tomography will facilitate and initiate other surgical procedures in the vicinity of the inner ear, such as facial canal repair and various
disorders in the otic capsule and inner ear meatus. It seems plausible that new
surgical procedures in the future will approach the inner ear walls as well as
structures in the inner ear compartments. We believe that such microsurgical
procedures have to be guided by preoperative radiographic information in
the same way as many other delicate neurosurgical operations.

References

ALTMANN, F. and ZECHNER, G.: The pathology and pathogenesis of endolymphatic hydrops.
    New investigations. Arch. klin. exp. Ohr.- Nas. KehlkHeilk. *192:* 1 (1968).
ANSON, B.J.: The endolymphatic and perilymphatic aqueducts of the human ear. Acta
    oto-lar. *59:* 140 (1965).
ARENBERG, I.K.; RASK-ANDERSEN, H.; WILBRAND, H., and STAHLE, J.: The surgical
    anatomy of the endolymphatic sac. Archs Otolar. *103:* 1 (1977a).
ARENBERG, I.K.; STAHLE, J.; WILBRAND, H.F., and NEWKIRK, J.B.: The unidirectional
    inner ear valve implant for endolymphatic sac surgery in Menière's disease. Archs
    Otolar. (submitted for publication, 1977b).
BRÜNNER, S. and PEDERSEN, C.B.: Experimental roentgen examination of the vestibular
    aqueduct. Acta radiol. *11:* 443 (1971).
CAWTHORNE, T.E. and HEWLETT, A.B.: Menière's disease. Proc. R.Soc. Med. *47:* 663 (1954).
CLEMIS, J.D. and VALVASSORI, G.E.: Recent radiographic and clinical observations on the
    vestibular aqueduct. Otolaryng. Clin. N. Am. *10:* 339 (1968).
ENANDER, A. and STAHLE, J.: Hearing in Menière's disease. A study of pure tone audio-
    grams in 334 patients. Acta oto-lar. *64:* 543 (1967).
GUSSEN, R.: Menière's disease. New temporal bone findings in two cases. Laryngoscope *81:*
    1695 (1971).
HALLPIKE, C.S. and CAIRNS, H.: Observations on the pathology of Menière's syndrome.
    J. Laryng. *53:* 625 (1938).
HARRISON, M.S. and NAFTALIN, L.: Menière's disease. Mechanism and management.
    American lecture series (Thomas, Springfield 1968).

MORRISON, A. W.: The surgery for vertigo. Saccus drainage for idiopathic endolymphatic hydrops. J. Laryng. *90:* 87 (1976).

ØIGAARD, A.; THOMSEN, J.; JENSEN, J., and DORPH, S.: The narrow vestibular aqueduct. An unspecific radiological sign? Archs Oto-Rhino-Laryng. *211:* 1 (1975).

PHELPS, P. D.: Paper read VIIth Cong. of Radiology in Oto-Rhino-Laryngology, Copenhagen 1976.

QUIST-HANSEN, S. and HAYE, R.: The natural course of Menière's disease. Acta Oto-Lar. (in press, 1976).

RASK-ANDERSEN, H.; SANDSTRÖM, B., and WILDBRAND, H. F.: The variational anatomy of the vestibular aqueduct (to be published, 1977).

RÖHLER, R.: Physiologische Probleme der Betrachtung des Röntgenbildes. Röntgenblätter *20:* 79 (1967).

RUMBAUGH, C. L.; BERGERON, T., and SCANLAN, R. L.: Vestibular aqueduct in Menière's disease. Radiol. Clins N. Am. *12:* 517 (1974).

SCHUKNECHT, H.: Pathology of the ear (Harvard University Press, Cambridge 1974).

SCHUKNECHT, H.: Discussion at the International Titisee Conference on 'Menière', 1976.

SHAMBAUGH, G. E.; CLEMIS, J. D., and ARENBERG, I. K.: Endolymphatic duct and sac in Menière's disease. Archs Otolar. *89:* 816 (1969).

SIEBENMANN, F.: Die Korrosions-Anatomie des menschlichen Ohres (Bergmann, Wiesbaden 1890).

STAHLE, J.: Electronystagmographic results in Menière's disease Otolaryng. Clin. N. Am. *10:* 509 (1968).

STAHLE, J.: Advanced Menière's disease. A study of 356 severely disabled patients. Acta oto-lar. *81:* 113 (1976).

STAHLE, J. and WILBRAND, H.: The vestibular aqueduct in patients with Menière's disease. A tomographic and clinical investigation. Acta oto-lar. *78:* 36 (1974a).

STAHLE, J. and WILBRAND, H.: The para-vestibular canaliculus. Can. J. Otolaryngol. *3:* 262 (1974b).

TUDDENHAM, W. J.: The visual physiology of roentgen diagnosis. A. Basic concepts. Am. J. Roentg. *78:* 116 (1957).

VALVASSORI, G. E.: L'aqueduc du vestibule et les affections du type vertigo de Menière. Traité Radiodiag. *17:* 355 (1974).

VALVASSORI, G. E.: Paper read VIIth Int. Cong. of Radiology in Oto-Rhino-Laryngology, Copenhagen 1976.

WILBRAND, H. F.: A tomographic test object. Acta radiol. *16:* 161 (1975).

WILBRAND, H. F.: Comparative anatomic and tomographic studies of the vestibular aquaeduct (to be published, 1977).

WILBRAND, H. F.; RASK-ANDERSEN, H., and GILSTRING, D.: The vestibular aqueduct and the para-vestibular canal. An anatomic and roentgenologic investigation. Acta radiol. *15:* 337 (1974).

WITTMAACK, K.: Die Ortho- und Pathobiologie des Labyrinthes (Thieme, Stuttgart 1956).

YUEN, S. S. and SCHUKNECHT, H. F.: Vestibular aqueduct and endolymphatic duct in Menière's disease. Archs Otolar. *96:* 553 (1972).

Doc. H. F. WILBRAND, Department of Diagnostic Radiology, Uppsala University Hospital, *S-750 14 Uppsala* (Sweden)

Adv. Oto-Rhino-Laryng., vol. 24, pp. 94–99 (Karger, Basel 1978)

Acoustic Neuromas Presenting with Symptoms of Morbus Menière

S. Grehn and J. Helms

Medizinisches Strahleninstitut (Direktor: Prof. W. Frommhold)
und Hals-Nasen-Ohren-Klinik (Direktor: Prof. D. Plester), Universität Tübingen, Tübingen

Progress in neurosurgical and otological microsurgery, especially the development of the translabyrinthine access with the aid of the operation microscope have made it possible to remove even small tumors within the internal auditory meatus with only low risk involved [4]. The adequate way for diagnosing such small neuromas is to perform a positive contrast cisternography in combination with multidirectional tomography [8]. This method leads to an exact diagnosis in respect to the location and the extent of such tumor. It offers the best information for the surgeon to decide whether or not the translabyrinthine approach to the tumor will be optimal for a successful treatment.

Our diagnostic procedure is as follows: After audiological, vestibular and neurological examinations the standard X-rays in Schüller's and Stenvers' projections are performed. As the first step to a more sophisticated examination the multidirectional tomography in a-p or if possible in p-a projection has to be done. By this means small differences in form and width of the internal auditory meatus can be observed as compared to the opposite side. This is very important, because only 27% of our patients having an acoustic tumor showed a unilateral enlargement of their meatuses of more than 7.5 mm in the standard films [1]. 29% had small differences that could only be detected in the tomograms. 44% did not show any difference in comparison to the opposite side. Even if these cases primarily present with symptoms of Menière's disease, the differential diagnosis of an acoustic neuroma has to be considered. As Plester [5] points out, the possibility has to be kept in mind that Menière's symptoms can be caused by an acoustic neuroma, whenever clinical, audiometric and vestibular signs are not equivocal.

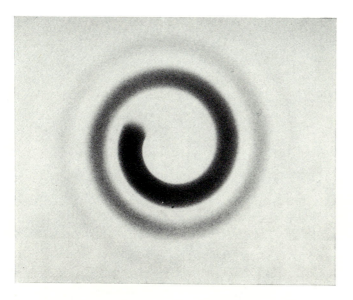

Fig. 1. All tomograms mostly have been performed in the spiral blurring of the Strato-matic.

Out of 44 acoustic tumors that have been seen in our hospital during the last 3 years, 3 had the typical symptoms of Menières disease, such as impairment of hearing, tinnitus and attacks of vertigo. Two more patients had a sudden deafness and this was the only symptom of their neuromas.

The best way of proving or excluding such tumors with atypical symptoms is to perform a positive contrast cisternography in combination with multi-directional tomography. The method of applicating the contrast medium and filling of the cerebellopontine angle cistern is well known [2, 3, 6].

We inject 1 ml of Duroliopaque to have a marking of the rim of the tumor only. Multidirectional tomography is of great advantage in order to see the real extent of the tumor without overlaying drops of the contrast medium. All tomograms have been performed in multidirectional blurring, a small number in the hypocycloidal form of the polytome or mostly – as the following examples – in the spiral blurring of the Stratomatic [7] (fig. 1).

Some examples may illustrate the radiological findings in the differential diagnosis of small acoustic neuromas.

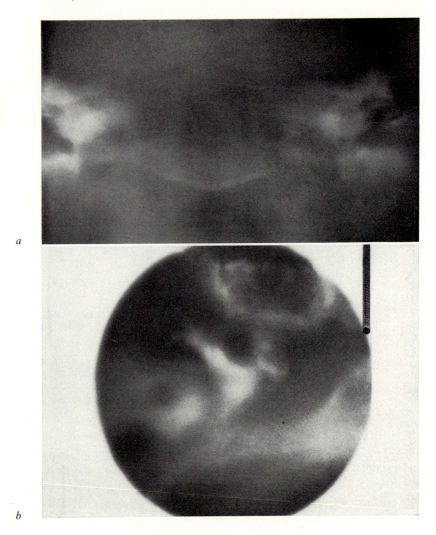

Fig. 2a, b. 39-year-old male with the typical symptoms and signs of Menière's disease. As conservative treatment had no effect, a positive contrast cisternography was performed prior to a planned saccotomy. This examination revealed a large, mainly extrameatal tumor of approximately 3 cm in diameter. No unilateral enlargement of one internal auditory could be seen.

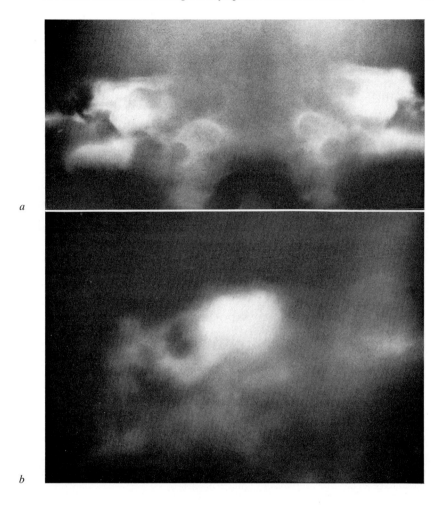

a

b

Fig. 3a,b. 68-year-old female with the typical symptoms of Menière's disease. A slight local enlargement of the right internal auditory meatus could be seen. The positive contrast cisternography revealed one of our smallest acoustic neuroma lying completely inside the meatus.

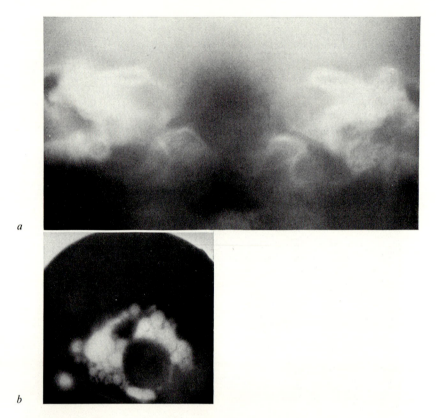

a

b

Fig. 4a, b. 55-year-old female who already underwent many neurological and otological examinations during the last 7 years because of a sudden deafness. Stenvers views, tomograms, angiograms and even a CT scan did not show any pathological findings. Finally a positive contrast cisternography was performed. This mainly extrameatally situated tumor proved to be an acoustic neuroma of 12 mm in diameter.

Summary

If a patient with Menière's disease or a sudden deafness does not respond to adequate therapy, an acoustic neuroma should be excluded. This is achieved by a positive contrast cisternography using multidirectional tomography. The examples might have shown that sometimes acoustic neuromas present with atypical symptoms, with sudden deafness or even with the typical symptoms of morbus menière.

References

1   BIEDERMANN, F. und LOEWE, G.: Die Varianten des Meatus acusticus internus. Bei-
    trag zur Röntgendiagnostik der Akustikusneurinome. Radiol.Diagn., Berlin 7: 141
    (1966).
2   CANIGIANI, G. und KNEISSEL, H.: Die positive Zisternographie in der Diagnostik der
    Kleinhirnbrückenwinkeltumoren. Mschr.Ohrenheilk.Lar.-Rhinol. 108: 28–33 (1974).
3   CAWTHORNE, T.: Diagnosis of acoustic neuroma. Archs Otolar. 89: 299 (1969).
4   FISCH, U. und Yasargil, M.G.: Der translabyrinthäre Zugang für die Akustikusneuri-
    nome. Practica oto-rhino-lar. 31: 111 (1969).
5   PLESTER, D.: Die Differentialdiagnose des Akustikusneurinoms. Dt.med.Wschr. 93:
    762 (1968).
6   VALVASSORI, G.E.: Diagnosis of acoustic neuromas. Archs Otolar. 89: 285 (1969).
7   VERGAU, W.; HEILMANN, H.P. und HELMS, J.: Tomographische Diagnostik des Felsen-
    beins mit spiraliger Verwischung. Fortschr.Roentgenstr. 116: 686 (1972).
8   WENDE, S. und NAKAYAMA, N.: Die neuroradiologische Diagnostik des Kleinhirn-
    brückenwinkeltumors. Z. Neurol. 203: 1 (1972).

Dr. S. GREHN, Medizinisches Strahleninstitut der Universität Tübingen, *Tübingen* (FRG)

Adv. Oto-Rhino-Laryng., vol. 24, pp. 100–105 (Karger, Basel 1978)

Abnormal Vestibular Aqueduct in Cochleovestibular Disorders

GALDINO E. VALVASSORI and JACK D. CLEMIS

Department of Radiology, University of Illinois,
and Department of Otolaryngology, Northwestern University, Chicago, Ill.

At the Symposium on Menière's Disease at Mayo Clinic in 1967 and several times afterwards, Dr. CLEMIS and I have reported on a clinical syndrome characterized by Menière-like disturbances and associated with a radiographically obliterated or abnormally filiform vestibular aqueduct.

Seven years later, at the Barany Society meeting in California, Dr. CLEMIS and I reported on the clinical findings and radiographic features of a congenital malformation characterized by a large vestibular aqueduct.

It is the purpose of this presentation to (1) review the radiographic features of these congenital or acquired abnormalities, (2) study their association with other anomalies of the inner ear structures, (3) analyze the clinical findings exhibited by patients with abnormal vestibular aqueducts, (4) attempt to correlate the clinical findings to the radiologic features.

Anatomy

The vestibular aqueduct is a bony canal in the otic capsule which extends from the medial wall of the vestibule to the outer opening in the posterior surface of the petrous pyramids and through which courses the endolymphatic duct.

In the fetus toward the mid-term the vestibular aqueduct has a straight course parallel to the common crus with the sac overlying the sigmoid sinus in the posterior fossa. The otic labyrinth reaches adult dimensions by mid-term, but growth and development of the structures of the posterior cranial fossa continue, resulting in a downward pull of the distal endolymphatic system by the sigmoid sinus and by the posterior fossa dura. This downward pull causes a change in the direction of the distal two-thirds of the vestibular aqueduct by bending it at a point just behind the common crus so that the aqueduct acquires its normal adult shape of an inverted 'J'.

The normal vestibular aqueduct in adults has an average length of approximately 10 mm and can be divided into two segments. The proximal segment or isthmus corresponding to the short limb of the 'J', has a length of approximately 1.5 mm and a mean diameter of 0.3 mm. The distal segment, which corresponds to the long limb of the 'J', is triangular in shape, with the apex at the junction with the isthmus and the base at the outer aperture. This segment is relatively capacious from side to side but compressed from top to bottom. At cross-section this segment is oval in shape with the largest diameter gradually increasing from 0.5 mm to over 5 mm at the external aperture. The short diameter ranges between 0.5 and 1.0 mm. In addition this segment undergoes a 20–30° torsion, imparting a propeller-like configuration.

Tomographic Technique

We have studied the vestibular aqueduct in a series of fresh temporal bones to select the best radiographic projection and to correlate the anatomical and radiographic findings. These bones were first tomographed in different planes and then sectioned after decalcification in one of the planes corresponding to the tomographic sections. From the previous anatomical description it became clear that the best views from the visualization of the vestibular aqueduct by tomography range from the lateral to the axial projection of the petrous pyramid. The direction and angle of rotation should be such as to turn the capacious side to side or transverse diameter of the aqueduct perpendicular to the plane of section and to align the outer opening of the aqueduct and the common crus in the same plane of section. From the practical point of view we usually start our study with a modified lateral projection obtained by rotating the petrous pyramid from the lateral 20° toward the axial projection. Sections are obtained 1 mm apart from the lateral end of the horizontal semicircular canal to the fundus of the internal auditory canal. If the vestibular aqueduct is not visualized or only partially seen, additional views are obtained in the straight lateral and/or axial projections. The distal segment of the aqueduct is usually well outlined, sectioned along its long axis. The proximal segment of the aqueduct, the isthmus, is instead quite often not detectable because of the narrowing of its lumen and because it becomes obscured by the contiguous common crus.

Control Study

The vestibular aqueduct was studied by tomography in 30 isolated temporal bones and in 100 consecutive cases with normal hearing or pure conductive loss. The segment of the vestibular aqueduct distal to the isthmus was satisfactorily visualized in one or more of the above described projections in all of the isolated temporal bones and in 92% of the cases. In the remaining 8%, the vestibular aqueduct was not clearly or only partially recognizable.

The isthmus of the aqueduct was clearly visible in only one third of the cases as it coursed to the vestibule underneath and parallel to the common crus.

Narrow Vestibular Aqueduct Syndrome

The selection of the cases was based on a complete or partial obliteration and narrowing of the vestibular aqueduct as detected by tomography. The determination of narrowing was based on the measurement of the aqueduct in the midpoint of the post-isthmic segment or half-way between the external aperture and the common crus. An aqueduct was considered narrowed whenever its anteroposterior diameter was less than 0.3 mm.

3000 consecutive cases referred for tomographic studies of the vestibular aqueduct because of cochleovestibular disorders were reviewed.

The symptomatology includes: (1) sensorineural hearing loss which may be reversible or fluctuant, progressive or irreversible; (2) tinnitus; (3) vertigo which may vary from severe type of whirling sensation associated with nausea and vomiting to mild positional vertigo; (4) fullness or pressure in the ear; (5) hyperacusis and diplacusis.

A normal visualization of both vestibular aqueducts was obtained in 1,715 cases (57%). One or both vestibular aqueducts were abnormal in 1,285 cases (43%). A more detailed breakdown of the patients with abnormal vestibular aqueduct is illustrated in table I.

When the clinical findings were correlated to the radiological features we found that the vestibular aqueduct was normal in most of the cases referred for sudden hearing loss or mild paroxysms of positional vertigo. A very high incidence of correlation was instead observed between radiographic nonvisualization or filiform aqueducts and clinical disturbances of the inner ear of the type of Menière's disease with abnormal audiometric and/or vestibular findings. It is particularly noteworthy that in patients in whom the non-visualization of the vestibular aqueduct was unilateral, we found a good

Table I. Abnormal vestibular aqueduct, 1,285 patients

Filiform and normal	290
Obliterated and normal	465
Total unilateral	755 (59%)
Filiform and filiform	115
Filiform and obliterated	140
Obliterated and obliterated	320
Total bilateral	485 (37.5%)
Large vestibular aqueducts	45 (3.5%)

correlation as far as the site of involvement in all instances but one. We also observed that several patients with unilateral inner ear symptomatology at the time of the tomographic study but bilateral nonvisualization of the aqueducts, later on developed similar findings in the opposite ear. Of course whereas the radiographic abnormalities of the vestibular aqueduct seem to correspond in a very high degree to otic pathology, normal visualization does not rule it out.

Large Vestibular Aqueduct Syndrome

The selection of the cases was based on an enlargement of the vestibular aqueduct as detected by tomography. Again the measurements of the aqueduct were obtained in the midpoint of the post-isthmic segment or half-way between the external aperture and the common crus. An aqueduct was considered enlarged whenever it's anteroposterior diameter was 1.5 mm or more. We reviewed in detail the tomographic and clinical findings of the first 30 consecutive cases.

The anteroposterior diameter of the enlarged vestibular aqueducts of the 30 cases under consideration ranged from 1.5 to 8 mm. The mean diameter was 4 mm. The anomaly was unilateral in 10 cases and bilateral in 20.

In 13 cases the only anomaly demonstrable by tomography was the enlarged vestibular aqueduct. Other anomalies of the labyrinth are probably present in these cases but limited to the membranous labyrinth and therefore not visible by radiographic means. In the other 17 cases the enlargement of the vestibular aqueduct was associated with anomaly of one or more of the inner ear structures.

The most common associated anomaly was an enlarged and rounded vestibule which was found in 13 of the patients. In 5 of these cases there was also an abnormal appearance of the semicircular canals, usually a dilatation of the ampullated portions of the horizontal and superior semicircular canals. In only one case was the vestibule hypoplastic: in the same case the semicircular canals were rudimentary and both cochleas and internal auditory canal considerably smaller than normal.

An abnormal appearance of the cochlea was found in 7 cases. In 6 cases the cochlea was hypoplastic and the bony partitions between the cochlear coils were deficient. In one case the cochlea was normal in size but there was no bony partition dividing the middle and apical coils.

The internal auditory canal was rarely involved: in only 1 instance was the canal hypoplatic and in 1 case abnormally large.

Of the 30 patients herein studied, 3 were referred for tomographic examination because of vestibular symptoms only. Radiographic abnormalities were confined to the vestibular aqueduct only in all 3 cases. Of the remaining 27 cases vestibular complaints could be elicited from many patients. Vestibular function tests were performed on only 4 patients and the responses were absent or markedly decreased in all instances. We may venture a suspicion, that vestibular responses would be abnormal in all cases of this series if this system was properly examined.

27 patients were referred for X-ray examination because of hearing losses. When the data could be classified, a pure tone sensorineural hearing loss was noticed in 30 ears, 13 bilateral and 4 unilateral problems. Mixed losses were noted in 19 ears. Three of the patients in the mixed group had undergone surgical exploration of the middle ear and in none was the reason of the conductive component identified. Fluctuation of hearing was recorded in 3 cases.

The age of onset could be traced to the first few years in life in at least two thirds of the cases. The anamnestic and radiographic information are certainly indicative of a congenital problem in most of the cases.

Conclusions

The tomographic evaluation of the vestibular aqueduct must be considered as a valid and valuable test in patients with cochleovestibular disorders. In an unselected series of 3,000 consecutive patients the vestibular aqueduct was abnormally narrow or obliterated in 41.5% and abnormally wide in 1.5%

of the cases. The radiographic information is not only interesting as a possible pathogenetic factor of endolymphatic hydrops but also important to the otologist in deciding when and how to attempt a surgical treatment.

G.E. VALVASSORI, MD, Professor, Department of Radiology, University of Illinois, *Chicago, Ill.* (USA)

Adv. Oto-Rhino-Laryng., vol. 24, pp. 106–114 (Karger, Basel 1978)

Nasal and Paranasal Sinus Polyposis

Current Concepts in Radiologic Diagnosis and Surgical Therapy

JUNE DEBOER UNGER, ROBERT J. TOOHILL, GEORGE F. UNGER
and OTTO F. GOMBAS

Departments of Radiology, Otolaryngology and Pathology, The Medical College
of Wisconsin, Milwaukee, Wisc., and the Radiology, Surgical and Laboratory
Services, Veterans Administration Center, Wood (Milwaukee), Wisc.

Introduction

Polypoid degeneration of the nasal and paranasal sinus mucosa is a
diesease entity which occurs in a significant number of the population and
produces distressing upper respiratory symptoms. During the past 5 years,
80 patients with this disorder have been surgically treated at our institutions.
Since all of these individuals were radiographically examined preoperatively
and a large number reexamined postoperatively, a wealth of clinical material
was made available to us. The purpose of this presentation is to state our
findings and discuss the method of radiologic investigation which we believe
provides optimal information.

Anatomical – Radiographic Considerations

Before proceeding with the main content of our material, which will
pertain primarily to the ethmoid sinuses, we would like to briefly discuss the
anatomy and radiography of this area.

The ethmoid bone is comprised of four parts: a horizontal or cribriform
plate, a perpendicular plate and two lateral masses or labyrinths. The average
adult measurements have been reported as 26.8 mm cephalocaudad, 32.7 mm
ventrodorsally and 14 mm mediolaterally [8]. It lies in direct relationship
with the anterior cranial fossa, medial orbital walls and nasal cavity, as well
as the frontal, maxillary and sphenoid sinuses.

The ethmoid air cells within the labyrinths may be divided into anterior and posterior groups according to drainage sites. The anterior cells drain into the middle meatus of the nose, whereas the posterior cells drain into the superior meatus. Middle ethmoidal cells are also described and located within a protuberance on the lateral nasal wall known as the ethmoidal bulla, but these may be appropriately considered with the anterior group because of similar drainage [4].

Agger cells may occur in any of the adjacent bony structures. Invasion of the middle turbinate is common and significant when polypoid degeneration is present.

The proximity of adjacent facial and cranial structures produces numerous interfering shadows on conventional radiographs. The two best views for visualization of the ethmoids are the PA or Caldwell and the oblique or Rhese projections. Some superimposition is still present, however, and occasionally diseased ethmoid sinuses may appear normal.

Etiology

The precise etiology of nasal and paranasal sinus polyposis is unclear, since no single factor has been found common to all patients [2,9]. There was proven allergy in approximately one-third of our cases. Although almost one-half of the patients used tobacco in some form, only a few were heavy smokers. A small number, who presented with rhinitis medicamentosa, were found to be either long-term users of topical nasal decongestants or on rauwolfia alkaloids for the treatment of systemic hypertension.

Infection, proven by culture, was present in over one-half of the patients and occasionally combined with allergy, vasomotor rhinitis or rhinitis medicamentosa.

Pathology

Chronic polypoid sinusitis is characterized by mucosal hypertrophy and hyperplasia, producing irregularities and crypts in the mucous membrane susfaces which predispose to further infection and inhibition of ciliary action. Retention cysts develop along with polypoid masses. The stromal tissue of the latter is markedly edematous and filled with inflammatory cells which may be predominately eosinophiles (fig. 1). Considerable vascular congestion is also present. These polyps may arise from the diseased mucosa anywhere

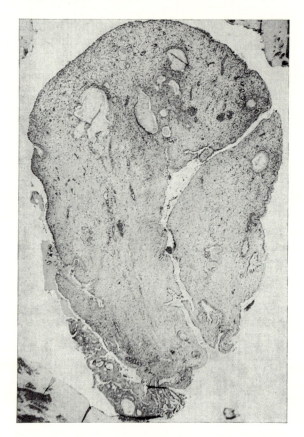

Fig. 1. Polyp removed during intranasal ethmoidectomy. The mucosa consists of pseudostratified ciliated respiratory epithelium and the underlying basement membrane is thickened and hyalinized. Marked edema of the stromal tissue is present and there are numerous inflammatory cells which are predominately eosinophils. Congested blood vessels are present. The cystic-appearing structures are actually dilated ducts lined with mucous-secreting cells.

in the nose or paranasal sinuses. Blockage of the draining ostia by intranasal polyps or those which arise from the sinus mucosa and protrude through the ostia into the nasal cavity is common.

Uncommon polypoid lesions which may present with a similar radiographic appearance include epithelial papillomas and inverting papillomas. The predisposition to malignant transformation of the epithelial papilloma can warrant a different surgical approach. Inverting papillomas are not a distinct pathologic entity but rather a morphologic variation which may

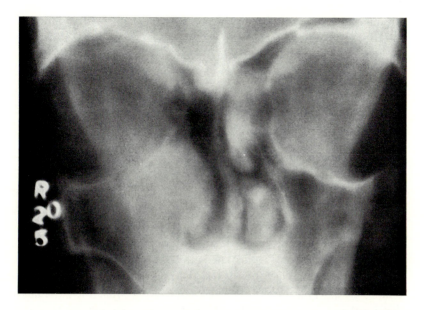

Fig. 2. Inverting papilloma. AP tomograms done 8 months postintranasal ethmoidectomy. A large mass is seen to protrude the right nasal cavity and the adjadent maxillary
antrum is opacified. The bony medial antral wall appears destroyed and there is thinning
and expansion of the inferomedial antral wall. At surgery the bony sinus walls, both
medially and anteriorly, were completely decalcified and generally unrecognizable. The
tumor was benign.

develop in ordinary nasal polyps or epithelial papillomas when invagination
of the surface epithelium occurs [1]. In one of our patients with an inverting
papilloma, however, there was substantial local bone resorption which radiographically and surgically resembled malignant invasion (fig. 2).

Surgery

Various surgical procedures have been utilized in the past for ameliora-
tion or cure of chronic nasal and paranasal sinus polyposis with varying
reports of success [3, 5, 7]. Intranasal ethmoidectomy, as performed here, is
usually done under local anesthesia with initial removal of gross nasal polypoid tissue and correction of nasal septal deviation, if necessary, to improve
surgical field exposure. The ethmoid labyrinth is entered through the bone of
the agger nasi of the ethmoidal bulla preceded by infracture of the middle

turbinate in order for this to be accomplished. All accessible anterior and posterior ethmoid cells are then carefully exenterated. During or following this procedure the middle turbinate is removed, both for purposes of exposure and to eliminate a locus for potential recurrence of disease. A middle meatal antrostomy is then performed in those patients with preoperative radiologic evidence of maxillary sinusitis [6].

Radiology

We initially reviewed the preoperative conventional paranasal sinus radiographs of 43 patients and were able to make a diagnosis of ethmoid disease in 39 by criteria which included mucosal thickening, fluid levels and partial or total opacification of air cells along with demineralization or obliteration of the bony septa. The paranasal sinus examinations appeared normal in the remaining 4 patients. There was evidence of other sinus disease in all 39 patients but only 7 exhibited pansinusitis, while the remainder had either isolated maxillary or frontal involvement or combined frontal and maxillary sinusitis which was occasionally unilateral (fig. 3). Definite polypoid change in the sinuses was apparent in only 2 patients, and we therefore concluded that sinus polyposis was generally radiographically indistinguishable from chronic sinusitis without polyposis. The presence of negative examinations in the 4 patients was disturbing, since there was significant disease present at surgery.

Since this original review was retrospective, it was decided to prospectively examine future patients using an established protocol which consisted of conventional sinus views (Caldwell, Walters, lateral, submentovertex and bilateral Rhese) and AP, lateral and submentovertex hypocycloidal tomography through the paranasal sinuses at 0.5-cm levels.

It soon became apparent that tomography provided even more information than anticipated (fig. 4). Polypoid sinus disease *per se* could be clearly demonstrated and diagnosed in all patients except those with total opacification secondary to ostia blockage. Xeroradiography was done on a few patients (fig. 5) to determine if the edge effect could produce enhancement of mucosal and bony structures, but did not provide any additional or even as much information as seen tomographically. We intend to further investigate this modality, but are limited at this time by radiographic tube heat tolerance.

23 of the original 43 patients were reexamined postoperatively by conventional radiography at intervals which varied from 2 to 5 years. Of these,

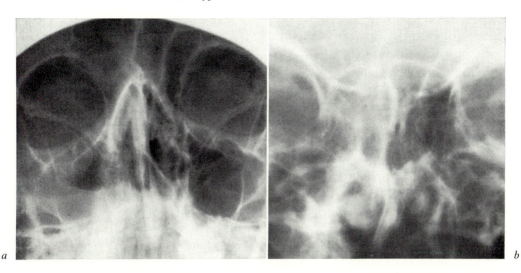

Fig. 3. a Water's view. Fluid levels are present in the right frontal and maxillary sinuses. *b* PA projection. The right ethmoid air cells appear uniformly opacified. Polypoid tissue is present in the upper portion of the right nasal cavity.

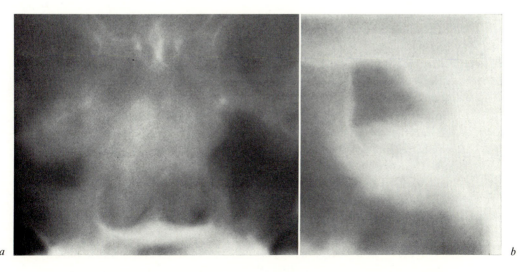

Fig. 4. a AP tomography. Multiple polyps are present in both maxillary antra and filling the upper halves of the nasal cavities. Uniform ethmoid opacification is present. *b* Lateral tomography. Polypoid tissue is present at the base of the sphenoid sinus.

ethmoid disease was present in 19 and absent in 4, appeared improved in 6 but unimproved or worse in comparison with the original studies in 14. No change was found in 3 patients. Since these positive findings correlated poorly with the generally good improvement or asymptomatic state of the patients, it was decided to also evaluate as many future postoperative patients as possible by tomography utilizing the same protocol as planned for the preoperative individual. It was hoped that by so doing the postoperative appearance could be established and serve as a criterion for evaluation of recurrence in the symptomatic postoperative patient. The initial examination is done 2 months after surgery, since regeneration of normal mucosa is expected by that time. The study is then repeated at 1- and 5-year intervals in the asymptomatic patients and, additionally, should symptoms reoccur at the time of recurrence.

These postoperative studies are providing an invaluable noninvasive means of exmining the sinus mucosa and have shown that definite disease, radiographically, may not actually represent recurrence of the original disease process or clinically significant disease (fig. 6).

Discussion

Intranasal ethmoidectomy, by the technique described above, appears to represent the procedure of choice in the treatment of severe chronic nasal and paranasal sinus polyposis. Clinical symptoms are primarily due to obstruction of the nasal fossae by polyps which arise from hypertrophied, diseased sinus mucosa and may prolapse through and occlude the sinus ostia. Relief of these symptoms occurs after polyp removal and ethmoid exenteration. Some degree of sinus disease frequently remains radiologically despite the fact that mucosal biopsy of the fovea ethmoidalis has revealed regeneration of normal mucosa.

Conventional radiography is generally inadequate in establishing the morphology and extent of disease, although this information is essential to the surgeon in making the decision to operate. Although these films may appear normal in symptomatic patients, we now know that pathology will probably be evident tomographically. Considering that a tenfold swelling of the lining mucosa is necessary to produce even a 1-mm visible width of mucosal edema [10], this is not surprising. Problems of superimposition noted above are eliminated by sectional radiography and even small fluid levels can be appreciated.

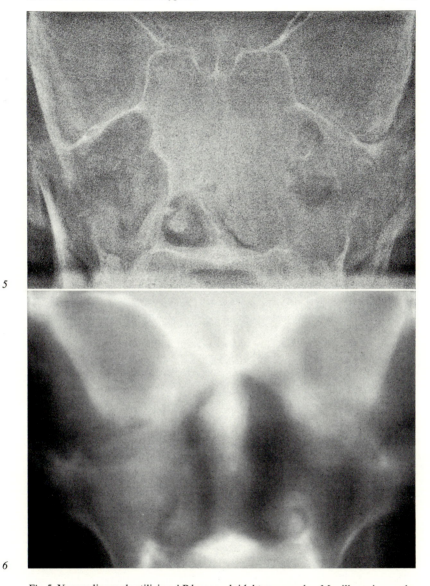

5

6

Fig.5. Xeroradiograph utilizing AP hypocycloidal tomography. Maxillary sinus polyposis may be seen along with ethmoid and nasal opacification. However, this film, done at the limit of tube tolerance, provided less detail than the corresponding AP tomogram.

Fig.6. AP hypocycloidal tomogram 2 months postintranasal ethmoidectomy. A few residual opacified ethmoid cells are seen. The right maxillary antrum is totally opacified and there is some mucosal thickening in the left maxillary antrum. Mucosal hypertrophy is seen along the nasal septum. The patient was totally asymptomatic.

Summary

We believe that hypocycloidal tomography is the method of choice in the pre- and postoperative evaluation of chronic nasal and paranasal sinus polyposis, based on the radiographic examinations of 80 patients who have undergone intranasal ethmoidectomy. Although our overall study is incomplete at this time due the extended period necessary for follow-up, we hops that the basic information which is now available will be beneficial to othere.

References

1   Anderson, W. A. D.: Pathology; 4th ed. p. 711 (Mosby, St. Louis 1961).
2   Davison, F. W.: Hyperplastic sinusitis – a five year study. Ann. Otol. Rhinol. Lar. *72:* 462–474 (1963).
3   Davison, F. W.: Intranasal surgery. Laryngoscope *79:* 502–511 (1969).
4   Eichel, B. S.: The intranasal ethmoidectomy procedure: historical, technical and clinical considerations. Laryngoscope *82:* 1806–1821 (1972).
5   Gray, H.: Anatomy of the human body; 29th American ed. pp. 180–183 (Lea & Febiger, Philadelphia 1973).
6   Kidder, T. L.; Toohill, R. J.; Unger, J. D., and Lehman, R. H.: Ethmoid sinus surgery. Laryngoscope *84:* 1525–1534 (1974).
7   Lillie, H. I. and Williams, H. L.: The external fronto-ethmosphenoid operation. Minn. Med. *18:* 786–789 (1935).
8   Schaeffer, J. P.: The nose and olfactory organ, pp. 205–233 (Blakiston, Philadelphia 1920).
9   Semenov, H.: The pathology of the nose and paranasal sinuses in relation to allergy. Trans. Am. Acad. Ophthal. Oto-lar. *56:* 121–170 (1952).
10 Semenov, H.: The surgical pathology of nasal sinusitis. J. Am. med. Ass. *111:* 2189–2195 (1938).

June D. Unger, MD, Radiology Service/114, Veterans Administration Center, *Wood, WI 53193* (USA)

Adv. Oto-Rhino-Laryng., vol. 24, pp. 115–142 (Karger, Basel 1978)

Calcifying and Osteoblastic Tumors of the Nasal and Paranasal Cavities

JUDAH ZIZMOR and ARNOLD M. NOYEK

Department of Radiology, New York University Medical Center, and Department Radiology, Manhattan Eye, Ear and Throat Hospital, New York, N.Y., and Department of Otolaryngology, University of Toronto Medical School, and Mount Sinai and Sunnybrook Hospitals, Toronto, Ont.

Calcifying and osteoblastic tumors of the paranasal sinus comprise a heterogeneous group of disorders characterized by certain correlating radiologic and pathologic features. The roentgen findings of macroscopic calcification, bone formation and bony reactive sclerosis in the paranasal sinuses are not often of themselves specific; however, a rather distinct group of diseases produce this group of radiologic signs, and therefore are readily considered in differential diagnosis. It is the purpose of this presentation to describe this group of calcifying and osteoblastic tumors. Space and time restrictions permit a selective rather than a total representation.

Calcifying and osteoblastic tumors of the paranasal sinuses and nasal cavities produce the following radiologic signs, singly or in combination: (1) calcification, (2) ossification, (3) one or more embryonic or fully developed teeth, and (4) osteoblastosis, hyperostosis and sclerosis.

Calcification and ossification cannot always be differentiated on X-ray examination. However, discernible bone texture indicates that bone formation has occurred. This may be quite obvious, or obscure in other instances. Secondary signs include encroachment of a calcific or osseous mass on adjacent sinus bony walls, decreased luminal volume of a sinus or nasal cavity and extrasinus extension into adjacent structures such as the orbits, nasal cavities, bony foramina, and intracranially.

A variety of pathogenic mechanisms produce calcification, ossification and osteoblastosis (table I). Within the tumor itself, parenchymal cells may calcify, or ossify. Calcification is, for example, particularly common in psammomatous meningioma. The rare formation of ossific phleboliths is almost pathognomonic for hemangiomas. Tumor stroma may also calcify, on a dystrophic rather than metastatic basis. Calcium deposition often occurs

Table I. Pathogenesis of calcific and osteoblastic radiologic signs

1	Intratumor	
	A Parenchyma	– calcification
		– ossification
		– tooth formation
	B Stroma	
2	Extratumor	– osteoblastosis
3	Combination	

Table II. Classification

I Calcifying and osteoblastic lesions simulating tumors
    a) Foreign body
    b) Osteoblastic osteomyelitis
    c) Calcifying polyps
    d) Calcifying mucoceles
    e) Bony dysplasia – e. g. fibrous dysplasia, Paget's disease
    f) Dental cysts – e. g. dentigerous cyst
    g) Other – Albers-Schönberg disease, lethal midline granuloma, reticuloses
       (regenerative phase)

II Calcifying and osteoblastic tumors
  A Benign
    1 Intrinsic
      a) Osteoma
      b) Chondroma and osteochondroma
      c) Hemangioma
      d) Miscellaneous – e. g. angiofibroma, mesenchymoma, benign osteoblastoma
    2 Extrinsic
      a) Dental – e. g. compound odontoma, complex odontoma
      b) Neurogenic tumors – e. g. meningioma, neurofibroma
      c) Miscellaneous – e. g. chordoma, craniopharyngioma

  B Malignant
    1 Primary
      a) Carcinoma – e. g. carcinoma nasopharynx
      b) Sarcoma – e. g. chondrosarcoma, osteogenic sarcoma
    2 Secondary
      a) Direct extension from adjacent structures – e. g. malignant mixed tumor,
        lacrimal gland
      b) Metastatic – e. g. carcinoma prostate

with trauma, inflammation, degeneration, necrosis and infarction of tissues. Bony reaction may occur about the margins of osteoblastic tumors, both benign and malignant. The benign tumor gives rise to a thin marginating regular line of sclerosis in most instances, whereas malignant tumor produces bone invasion with a more dense irregular poorly defined zone of sclerotic reactivity [11]. Combinations of both intratumor and extratumor calcification and osteoblastosis may occur, as in chordoma.

The following classification (table II) of calcifying and osteoblastic tumors affords an understandable presentation.

I. Calcifying and Osteoblastic Lesions Simulating Tumors

The majority of foreign bodies occur in the nasal cavities and are termed rhinoliths. These calcify by precipitation of calcium salts, and serve as a nidus for accumulation of inspissated secretions and may form a pseudo-tumor mass. Foreign bodies also occur within the maxillary sinus. These are termed antroliths (fig. 1). Many of these may calcify, whether of exogenous or endogenous origin; the most common foreign body is dental or dental-related.

Of the inflammatory diseases, osteomyelitis is the most productive of osteoblastosis (Garrés sclerosing osteomyelitis). Osteoblastic osteomyelitis (fig. 2) represents an exuberant reparative phase in the inflammatory process, either bacterial or fungal in origin. The production of bony sequestra may add to the hyperostotic roentgen appearance of these lesions.

Chronic hypertrophic polypoid disease involving the nasal mucosa and paranasal sinus mucosa, represents a localized response to systemic allergy. However, nasal and sinus polyps in rare instances may calcify and may produce both displacement and erosion of bony walls (fig. 3). Proptosis may result from an expanding benign ethmoidal polypoid lesion eroding intraorbitally. This polypoid lesion may calcify and simulate a mucocele or tumor invading the orbit.

In a comprehensive review of mucocele cases [28], it has been noted that 5% of mucoceles demonstrate macroscopic calcification, detectable on X-ray examination. In some instances the calcification may be sufficiently dense to simulate an osteoma, usually of the frontal sinus (fig. 4).

Though dental cysts, such as the radicular cyst, do not usually calcify, dystrophic calcification can occur within the cyst wall if a long-standing inflammatory reaction is present. The most constantly observed calcific or

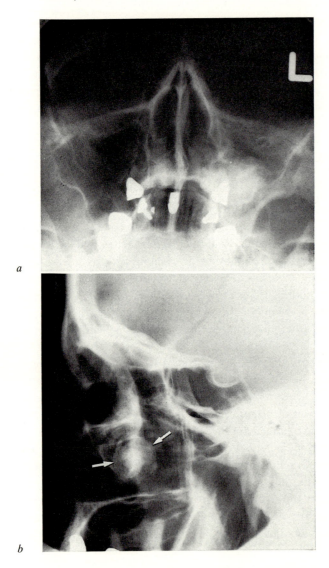

Fig. 1. Antrolith, left maxillary sinus. *a* A Waters view demonstrates a partly calcified soft tissue mass occupying the lower two thirds of the left maxillary sinus. The mucous membrane of the maxillary sinus is moderately increased. *b* A lateral view demonstrates lamellated calcification in the antrolith (arrows). From ZIZMOR and NOYEK [33].

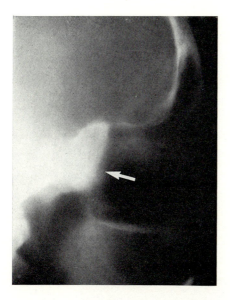

Fig. 2. Chronic osteoblastic osteomyelitis, sphenoid sinus. A lateral tomogram demonstrates obliteration of the sphenoid sinus lumen by secondary chronic sclerosing osteolitis with hyperostotic bone formation (arrow). The sphenoid sinus has been the site of a chronic suppurative sinusitis, which eventuated in osteomyelitis with osteoblastosis. This is an unusual radiographic finding in this area, and must be differentiated from primary osteoblastic tumors such as meningioma and prostatic metastasis. From ZIZMOR and NOYEK [33].

ossific density in relation to dental cysts is the presence of a tooth, either in whole or in part (fig. 5a, b), located at the periphery of a dentigerous cyst [27]. A dentigerous cyst results if cystic degeneration occurs in the dental bud after formation of enamel and dentin from epithelial and mesenchymal precursors, prior to the stage of eruption. Clinically, a missing tooth is noted in the dental arch, accompanied by the characteristic roentgen signs noted; this allows differentiation from the primordial or follicular cyst, in which differentiation of dental elements does not occur. Dentigerous cysts occur more commonly in the mandible than the maxilla; however, their importance is heightened by the fact that the aggressive ameloblastoma may arise from a preexisting dentigerous cyst.

The group of bone dysplasias can give rise to osteoblastosis sufficient to simulate tumor [6, 26]. Fibrous dysplasia may commonly simulate neoplastic disease, especially if the lesion has the characteristics termed by the

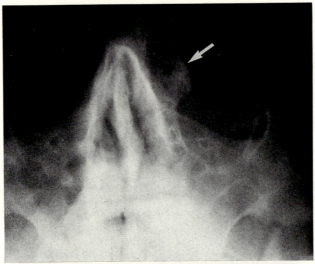

3

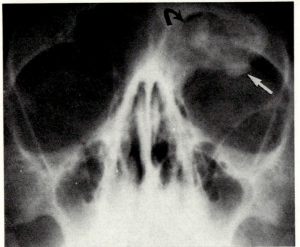

4

Fig.3. Calcified ethmoid polyps. A Waters view demonstrates a calcified cluster of ethmoidal polyps (arrow) which have extended into the left orbit producing exophthalmos in a 56-year-old man. The left maxillary sinus is completely opacified by thickened mucosa, and polypoid changes in the mucous membrane of the right maxillary sinus are also seen. From ZIZMOR and NOYEK [26, pp. 459–472].

Fig.4. Heavily calcified left frontal sinus mucocele. A Waters view demonstrates a heavily calcified frontal mucocele involving the left frontal sinus, simulating an osteoma (white arrow). Note the smooth bone erosion of the roof of the frontal sinus medially, as well as the sclerosis in the adjacent bone, often associated with mucocele (curved black arrow). From ZIZMOR and NOYEK [27].

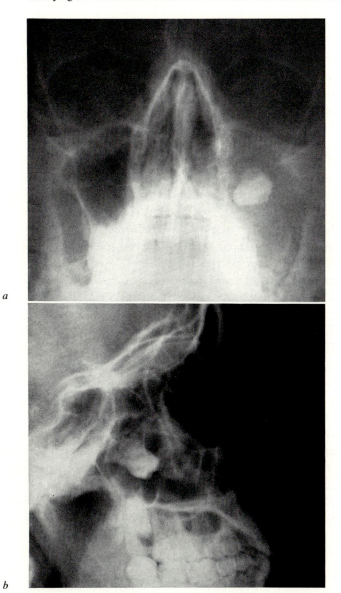

Fig. 5. Dentigerous cyst, left maxillary sinus. *a* A Waters view demonstrates an opaque left maxillary antrum as well as a smooth dehiscence of the left lateral antral wall. A dental crown is apparent within the antral mass. *b* A lateral view confirms the presence of a dentigerous cyst with a dental crown pointing downward and centrally from its attachment below the orbital floor posteriorly. From ZIZMOR and NOYEK [33] and courtesy Dr. J. STUCKLER, Toronto.

pathologist as ossifying fibroma. Fibrous dysplasia [14,15,19] is, in fact, a nonneoplastic disorder produced by bony overgrowth and deformity, due to a maturational arrest at the woven bone stage in intramembranous ossification [24]. Lamellar bone does not usually form. Ossifying fibroma [25] reflects the appearance of osteoblasts within the lesion, and subsequent bone formation. The practical importance of this radiologic-pathologic correlation lies in the fact that ossifying fibroma is more amenable to surgical resection than fibrous dysplasia (fig. 6a, b).

Generally, fibrous dysplasia occurs in monostotic, regional or generalized forms. The generalized form may be associated with a variety of endocrine changes, such as Albright's syndrome of precocious puberty [1]. The grotesque facial deformity which results from fibrous dysplasia, in most instances, is termed leontiasis ossea. However, the leontiasis deformity is not specific for fibrous dysplasia alone. Conservative surgical measures are indicated to alleviate deformity and nerve compression.

Paget's disease (osteitis deformans) produces replacement of normal bone by expanded soft osteoid and poorly mineralized bone. Of itself, it does not simulate tumor; however, it is felt that approximately 5% of cases of Paget's disease may eventuate in osteogenic sarcoma, which can be recognized by either bone destruction, or in some instances, calcification and bone formation. A variety of disorders complete the miscellaneous group. Albers-Schönberg disease [16] (fig. 7) is a rare disorder inherited as a Mendelian recessive, affecting both sexes equally. There is a marked bony overgrowth and sclerosis, sufficient to produce obliteration of marrow cavities and encroach on foramina. It affects the axial skeleton, ribs, long bones and skull base. Occasional sinus involvement is noted, and such a case is demonstrated. Lethal midline granuloma may rarely calcify and induce osteoblastosis, either in isolated form or as part of Wegener's granulomatosis spectrum of disease. The reticuloses usually do not calcify or produce bone reaction; however, successful treatment is often accompanied by both calcification and bony healing. The healing reaction may be sufficient to induce marked sclerosis.

Fig.6. Fibrous dysplasia, left maxillary sinus. *a* A Waters view demonstrates the typical findings of mixed ossific and fibrous expansion and obliteration of the left maxillary sinus lumen, due to fibrous dysplasia. There is expansion of its lateral and medial walls, as well as its roof (arrow) producing exophthalmos. *b* A lateral view demonstrates focal areas of calcification and ossification within the mass, as well as elevation of the orbital floor (arrow). Fibrous dysplasia may be termed ossifying fibroma once bone maturation occurs within the lesion. From ZIZMOR and NOYEK [29].

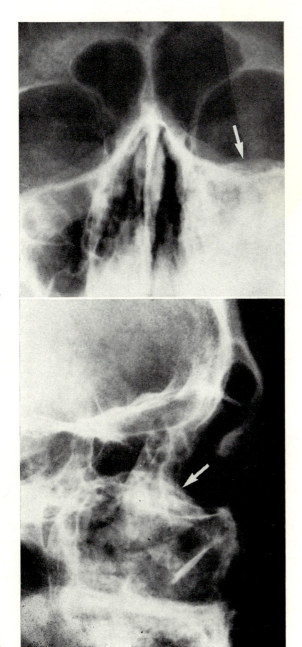

a

b

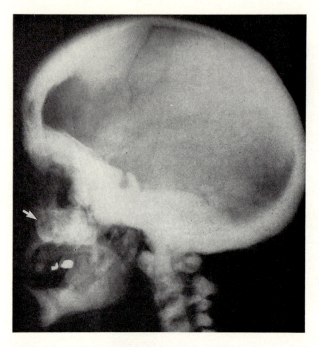

Fig. 7. Alber's-Schönberg disease (osteopetrosis), involving maxillary sinuses. A lateral view of the skull demonstrates homogeneous hyperostotic bony thickening of the base of the skull, which obliterates the sphenoid sinuses and thickens the sellar bony walls. Platybasia is also present. Bony thickening dents the outlines and obliterates the superimposed maxillary antra (arrow). The frontal bone, mandible and cervical spine are also involved. From ZIZMOR and NOYEK [32].

II. Calcifying and Osteoblastic Tumor

A. Benign [7, 26]

1. Intrinsic

Osteoma [17b, 27] is the most common of the intrinsic group of calcifying and osteoblastic tumors. In fact, it is the most common of all mesenchymal tumors of the paranasal sinuses. Osteoma, frequently found on incidental roentgen examination in the absence of symptoms, has a predilection for the frontoethmoid suture. Osteoma is described in two pathologic forms, though a variety of descriptive terms are used for these lesions. The hard, cortical, ivory or lamellar osteoma (fig. 8) is contrasted with the soft, cancellous or mature osteoma (fig. 9) or mixed osteoma (fig. 10). It should be noted that

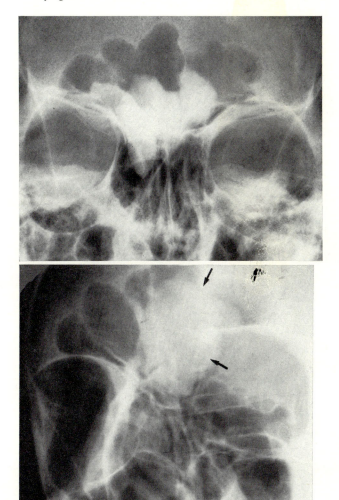

8

9

Fig. 8. Cortical osteoma, both frontal sinuses. A Caldwell view demonstrates the typical lobulated appearance of an ivory-dense frontal sinus osteoma, which appears to have arisen within the right frontal sinus at the region of the frontoethmoid suture line and expanded into the left frontal sinus. It also appears to extend into the ethmoid air cell system. The nasofrontal duct is presumably patent, as both frontal sinuses remained aerated. The cortical osteoma is also termed a hard osteoma, from the clinical point of view. From ZIZMOR and NOYEK [33].

Fig. 9. Cancellous osteoma, left frontal sinus. A left orbital oblique view shows a soft or cancellous osteoma filling the lower two-thirds of the left frontal sinus and blocking the nasofrontal duct. Note clouding of the frontal sinus by retained secretions. Its relationships are well shown in this view (arrows).

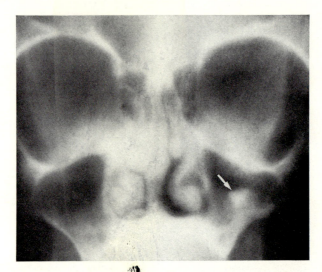

Fig. 10. Mixed hard and soft osteoma, left maxillary sinus. A coronal tomogram demonstrates a small mixed osteoma arising from the inferolateral wall of the left maxillary sinus, post Caldwell-Luc surgery. From Noyek *et al.* [17b].

osteomas may be multiple and may expand both extracranially and intracranially (fig. 11a, b). Multiple osteomas may form part of the complex of Garnder's syndrome [8] (fig. 12), in which there is an association with multiple polyposis of the colon and a tendency of these to undergo malignant denereration.

Chondroma [4, 21] is a very rare mesenchymal tumor which produces calcification in just over half of cases (fig. 13a). These calcifications may be either fine or coarse, and portions of the chondroma may ossify, producing a variety of pathologic descriptions such as osteochondroma or osteochondromyxoma. Benign osteoblastoma and mesenchymoma (fig. 13b) are also encountered.

Hemangioma of the paranasal sinuses rarely produces characteristic pheboliths (fig. 14) but hemangiomas undergoing clotting may calcify and ossify producing these concretions. Its recognition is surgically important, as it allows for angiographic evaluation and appropriate surgical measures, or the use of other treatment modalities such as embolization. Hemangioma of the paranasal sinuses usually involves the maxillary antrum, and has a predilection to increase rapidly in size during adolescence and pregnancy.

Rarely, a hemangioma of the nasal bones may be seen. When encountered, it is usually a lytic honeycombed lesion. However, we have seen fine trabecular calcifications extending beyond the confines of the nasal bones in the presence

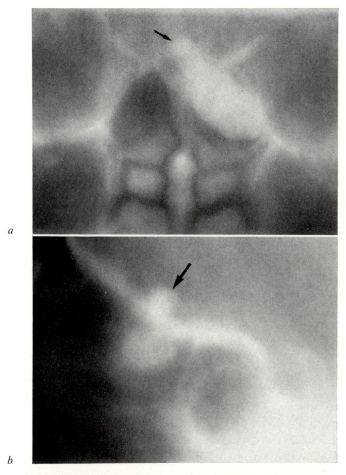

Fig. 11. Ethmoid osteoma with intracranial extension. *a* A coronal tomogram demonstrates a small osteomatous projection into the floor of the anterior cranial fossa (arrow) from a large lobulated osteoma occupying the left ethmoid labyrinth. *b* A lateral tomogram defines the anteroposterior dimension of the projection intracranially (arrow). The patient is a 19-year-old female. From ZIZMOR and NOYEK [32].

of hemangioma, and this would seem to be an unusual but unique, and diagnostic, finding. Such a case is illustrated in figure 15a and b.

A heterogenous group of benign mesenchymal tumors may also produce calcification or osteoblastosis. Angiofibroma, the second most common of all mesenchymal tumors, an important aggressive lesion of adolescent males, may induce sclerosis on some occasions. Sclerotic reaction occurs in the region of the pterygoid plates, in conjunction with anterior bowing of the posterior wall

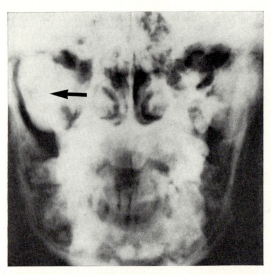

Fig. 12. Gardner's syndrome. A Caldwell view demonstrates a large osteoma involving the lateral wall of the right maxillary antrum (arrow); several small osteomas are present in the left maxillary sinus as well.

of the maxillary sinus. Related signs may be lucency of the sphenoid sinus with marginal osteoblastosis and enlargement of the lower outer margin of the superior orbital fissure.

2. Extrinsic

Among the dental tumors [10], those of epithelial origin with inductive connective tissue changes may present diagnostic radiologic features. The compound odontoma is demonstrated radiologically by the elements resulting from the differentiation of epithelial and mesenchymal precursors into enamel, dentin, cementum and pulp components [27]. Fully formed teeth may be evident within the tumor, as well as myriads of tiny embryonic teeth termed denticles (fig. 16a, b). Denticles have been noted in the hundreds, with as many as 2,000 having been described in one instance.

The complex odontoma is somewhat less common than the compound odontoma, and presents radiologically as an amorphous mass of undifferen-

Fig. 13. a Chondroma sphenoid sinus. A lateral tomographic view of the sphenoid sinus and sella turcica demonstrates the destruction of the sellar floor and dorsum sellae, as well as the posterior clinoid processes by a chondroma which invades the sphenoid sinus (arrow) and occupies its posterior half. Several areas of calcification are noted in the tumor, suggesting its pathologic nature. From ZIZMOR and NOYEK [33]. *b* Mesenchymoma of naso-

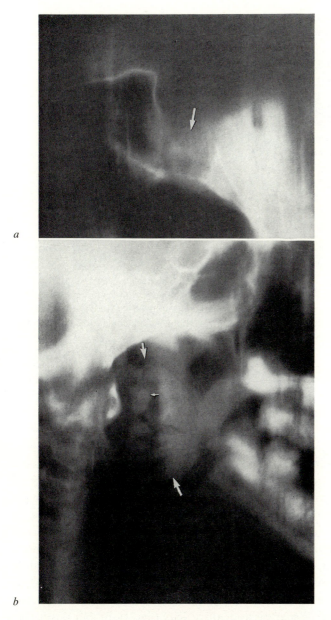

a

b

pharynx. A lateral tomogram of the nasopharynx demonstrates a large egg-shaped mass (large arrows) which prolapses into the nasopharynx in a 7-year-old boy. The entire post-nasal airway is obstructed. Several large calcific densities (tiny arrow) are seen within the tumor mass. From ZIZMOR and NOYEK [33] and courtesy Dr. D. MITCHELL, Toronto.

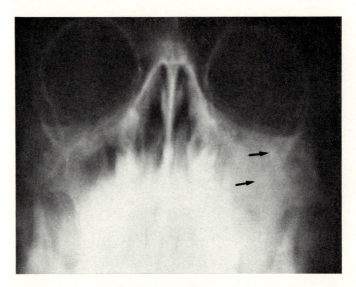

Fig. 14. Hemangioma, left maxillary sinus. A Waters view indicates opacification of the left maxillary sinus by a soft tissue mass which has eroded its lateral wall. There are several phleboliths in the mass, diagnostic of cavernous hemangioma (arrows). Courtesy Dr. E. AFSHANI, Buffalo, N.Y.

tiated calcific elements (fig. 17). Ameloblastoma is not a calcifying tumor of itself, and usually produces a destructive osteolytic appearance; however, as it may arise from a preexisting dentigerous cyst, a tooth may be noted within the expansile destructive lesion (fig. 18). A cementifying fibroma is shown in figure 19.

Neurogenic tumors comprise an important group of calcifying and osteoblastic neoplasma. Meningioma [9] is the most important in this group, as it comprises approximately 15% of all brain tumors. 20% of all meningiomas arise in a parasagittal position, in relation to the sphenoid (fig. 20a, b), ethmoid and frontal sinuses. Meningioma characteristically expands and compresses structures, but it may also be flat and spreading, producing a meningioma 'en plaque'. The tumor [12] not only calcifies, it may produce gross enostosis, a diagnostic feature. It may also initiate a dense osteoblastic reaction, often simulating the en plaque appearance of a meningioma proper.

The neurofibroma may occasionally calcify (fig. 21a, b), but this is very uncommon. Generally, calcification within a neurofibroma suggests a search for systemic neurofibromatosis. Chordoma [2, 3, 21] may calcify and contain sequestered destroyed bone. Its usual origin is from the clivus, in which case it

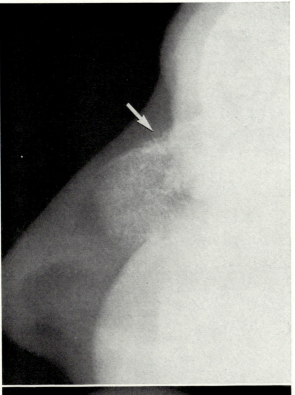

a

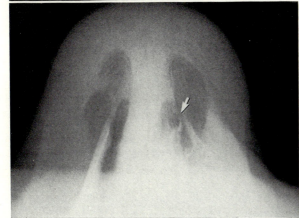

b

Fig. 15. Hemangioma, left nasal bone. *a* A lateral view of the nasal bones demonstrates
a bizarre net-like texture involving the left nasal bone. Peripheral spiculation associated
with osteoblastosis involves the upper half of the nasal bone towards the dorsum (arrow).
The osteoblastosis and bone texturing are typical of nasal bone hemangioma. *b* A supero-
inferior axial view demonstrates the findings confined to the left nasal bone (arrow). From
ZIZMOR and NOYEK [33].

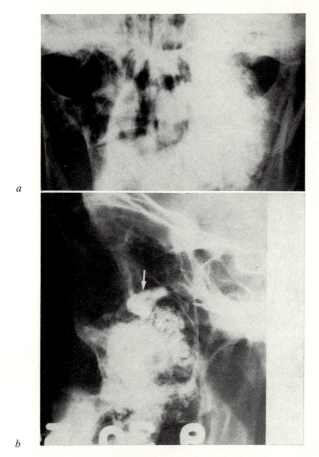

Fig. 16. Compound odontoma, left maxillary sinus. *a* A Caldwell view demonstrates a calcareous mass filling the left maxillary sinus. *b* A lateral view demonstrates the radiographic findings in a huge compound odontoma involving the maxillary sinus. The mass extends upwards into the orbit, elevating its floor by a single well-formed tooth (arrow). The remainder of the giant calcareous mass demonstrates differentiation into myriads of denticles (embryonic teeth). From ZIZMOR and NOYEK [27].

produces both bone destruction and dense retrosellar calcification, sometimes destroying the sphenoid sinus. Ectopic chordoma within the paranasal sinuses can occur. Craniopharyngioma [21] is usually recognized by its universal calcification. It arises in the craniopharyngeal duct from epithelial cells passing through the sphenoid bone in pituitary embryology. Cystic tumors usually produce curvilinear calcifications; though its usual extension is suprasellar, it can extend into the sphenoid sinus.

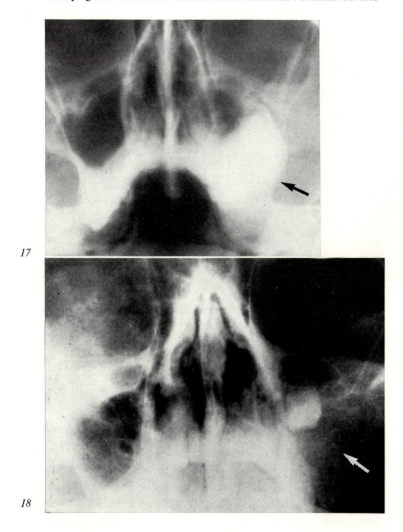

17

18

Fig. 17. Complex odontoma, left maxillary antrum. A Waters view indicates a dense calcific mass filling most of the left maxillary sinus in its outer portion. The inferolateral wall is slightly displaced externally (arrow). Complex odontoma is less common than compound odontoma, and fails to demonstrate differentiated elements in enamel and dentin formation. It simulates an osteoma. From ZIZMOR and NOYEK [30].

Fig. 18. Ameloblastoma, left maxillary sinus. A Waters view demonstrates destruction of the inferolateral antral wall on the left (arrow) along its entire length, by a soft tissue mass arising from the upper alveolus. A tooth is noted within the mass, representing the infrequent instance in which an ameloblastoma arises in a preexisting dentigerous cyst. From ZIZMOR and NOYEK [31].

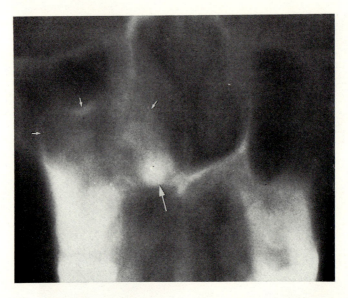

Fig. 19. Cementifying fibroma, right maxillary sinus. A coronal tomogram of the right maxillary sinus demonstrates a cementifying fibroma of the right upper alveolus extending into the right antrum and encroaching on the right nasal cavity. The large arrow indicates a dental crown at the inferomedial aspect of the mass. The numerous fibrous and calcific foci indicate a possible relationship with fibrous dyplasia. From ZIZMOR and NOYEK [30].

B. Malignant

1. Primary

The only carcinoma in which sclerosis may be an anticipated roentgen finding is carcinoma of the nasopharynx. This disease has a predilection for southern Chinese. Sclerosis [18, 23] is an uncommon radiologic feature as the tumor involves the vault of the nasopharynx, base of skull, and related paranasal sinus and other structures. It was once felt that this sclerotic reaction was typical of the so-called transitional cell carcinoma, but it is now recognized by electron microscopic studies that transitional cell carcinoma is, in fact, an undifferentiated squamous cell carcinoma; the tonofibrils of squamous epithelium can be demonstrated. The osteoblastic variant of this tumor is rare. It may be encountered in children as well as in adults.

Carcinoma of the nasopharynx may extend into the middle fossa and obliterate foramina and involve other basal skull structures such as the pterygoid plates in dense osteoblastic reaction (fig. 22a–c). Radiotherapy may also promote similar osteoblastosis.

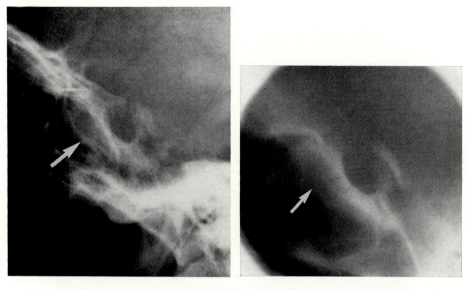

Fig. 20. Osteoblastic meningioma, invading sphenoid sinus. *a* A lateral view demonstrates an osteoblastic mass occupying the upper half of the sphenoid sinus (arrow). *b* A lateral tomogram further defines the bony meningiomatous plaque as it extends from the sella into the sphenoid sinus. Further studies with angiography and computed tomography demonstrated narrowing of the internal carotid artery and the extent of intracranial component of the tumor. From NOYEK *et al.* [17a].

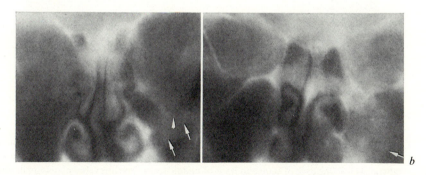

Fig. 21. Neurofibroma, left maxillary sinus. *a* An A-P tomogram demonstrates a soft tissue density occupying the upper medial portion of the left maxillary sinus (arrows). It erodes the inferomedial wall of the left infraorbital canal (arrowhead), producing intractable pain in the left cheek. *b* An A-P tomogram more posteriorly demonstrates the tumor mass (arrow), with numerous areas of pinpoint calcific foci within it. From ZIZMOR and NOYEK [33].

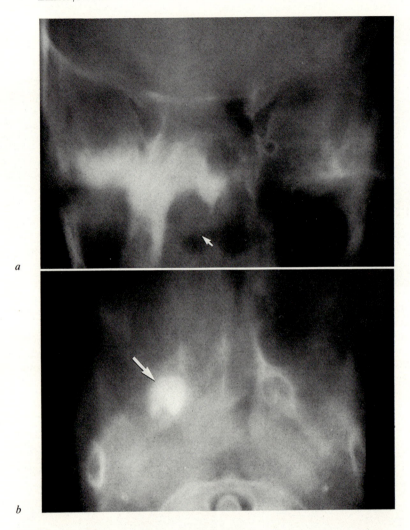

a

b

Fig. 22. Carcinoma of the nasopharynx with bone sclerosis. *a* A coronal tomogram demonstrates a dense osteoblastic reaction involving the sphenoid sinus margins on the right, as well as the base of skull and floor of middle fossa. The pterygoid plates are densely thickened by osteoblastic reaction, secondary to an infiltrating carcinoma of the nasopharynx. The arrow demonstrates a soft tissue mass prolapsing into the postnasal airway. *b* A basal tomogram defines the osteoblastosis involving the pterygoid plates (arrow) as compared with the opposite side. *c* A lateral tomogram defines the A-P dimension of the osteoblastic reaction to a squamous cell carcinoma of the nasopharynx in a young southern Chinese adult female.

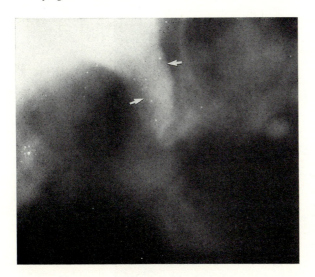

c

Chondrosarcoma may demonstrate fine to coarse calcification in approximately one third of cases. Its usual radiologic sign is an expanding soft tissue mass. Calcification often increases following radiotherapy, and the disease may run an exceedingly long course (fig. 23a, b).

Osteogenic sarcoma may also calcify or produce bone, either as ray-like spicules (fig. 24) or dense clumps of bone formation (fig. 25). This is a relatively infrequent occurrence. Previous radiotherapy to bone or preexisting fibrous dysplasia or Paget's disease of bone increases the incidence of osteogenic sarcoma.

2. Secondary [5]

Direct extension of calcifying or ossifying malignant tumors into the sinus is unique; such a case is shown involving a malignant mixed tumor of the right lacrimal gland extending to the right frontal sinus (fig. 26).

Carcinoma of the prostate [20,22] is the only documented tumor to produce osteoblastic metastases to the skull and paranasal sinuses with regularity (fig. 27). Some metastatic prostatic lesions produce lysis or bone destruction and bone production simultaneously. Carcinoma of the prostate metastasizes via the paravertebral veins of Batson and exhibits a predilection for metastasis to the axial skeleton and skull base and allied paranasal sinuses. The dense osteoblastosis [13,22] is a reaction to the invasion of Haversian systems by tumor cells. Successful endocrine therapy may convert osteolytic metastases to osteoblastic lesions.

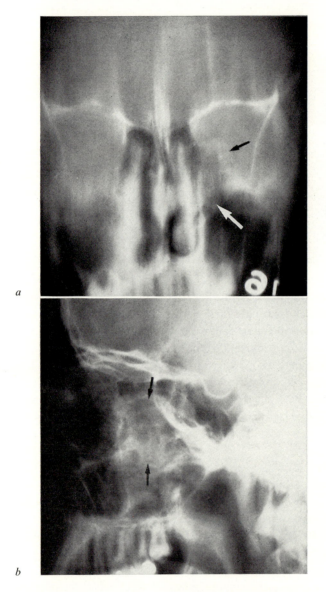

a

b

Fig. 23. Chondrosarcoma, ethmoid sinus. *a* A coronal tomogram demonstrates a soft tissue mass with small calcific foci arising within the left ethmoid labyrinth and invading the orbit and prelacrimal recess of the left maxillary sinus. *b* A lateral view demonstrates the calcific foci evident within the soft tissue mass (arrows). From ZIZMOR and NOYEK [33] and courtesy Dr. W.S. GOODMAN, Toronto.

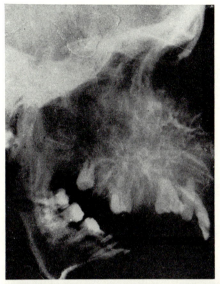

24

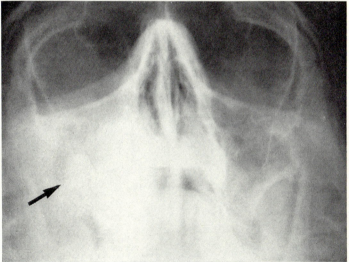

25

Fig. 24. Osteogenic sarcoma, maxillary sinus. A lateral radiograph demonstrates a huge osteogenic sarcoma of the right maxillary sinus which has entirely destroyed the upper jaw and hard palate. It extends superiorly into the orbit and posteriorly. The bony spiculations in such a destructive lesion are virtually diagnostic of osteogenic sarcoma. From ZIZ-MOR and NOYEK [26] and courtesy Dr. L. HIRANANDANI, Bombay, India.

Fig. 25. Osteogenic sarcoma, left maxillary sinus. A Waters view demonstrates an opacified right maxillary sinus with osseous foci (arrow). There is destruction of the infero-lateral wall of the maxillary sinus. Courtesy Dr. G. WORTZMAN, Toronto, Canada.

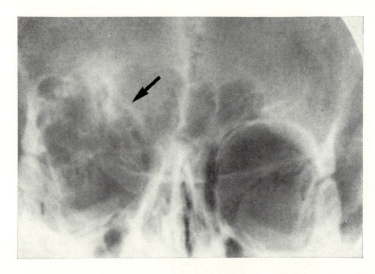

Fig. 26. Malignant mixed tumor, right lacrimal gland extending into right frontal sinus. A mixed osteolytic and osteoblastic lesion has destroyed the roof of the right orbit and the lacrimal fossa. It extends into the lateral aspect of the frontal sinus (arrow). The floor of the frontal sinus is eroded on this side. This proved to be a malignant mixed tumor of the lacrimal gland. From ZIZMOR and NOYEK [32].

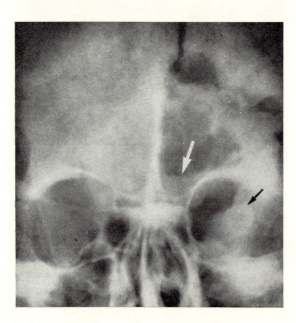

References

1 ALBRIGHT, F.; BUTLER, A.M.; HAMPTON, A.O., and SMITH, P.: Syndrome characterized by osteitis fibrosa disseminata, areas of pigmentation and endocrine dysfunc-
   tion with precocious puberty in females. New Engl.J.Med. 216: 727–746 (1937).

2 BATSAKIS, J.G. and KITTLESON, A.C.: Chordomas. Archs Otolar. 78: 168–175 (1963).

3 BERDAL, P. and MYRHE, E.: Cranial chordomas involving the paranasal sinuses. J.
   Laryng. 78: 906–919 (1964).

4 BERKMEN, Y.M. and BLATT, E.S.: Cranial and intracranial cartilaginous tumors. Clin.
   Radiol. 19: 327–333 (1968).

5 COPELAND, M.M.: Metastases to bone from primary tumours in other sites. Proc.
   natn. Cancer Conf. 6: 743–756 (1970).

6 FRIES, J.W.: Roentgen features of fibrous dysplasias of skull and facial bones. Am.J.
   Roentg. 77: 71–88 (1957).

7 FU, Y.-S. and PERZIN, K.H.: Non-epithelial tumours of the nasal cavity, paranasal
   sinuses and nasopharynx: a clinico-pathologic study. Cancer 33: 1289–1305 (1974).

8 GARDNER, E.J. and RICHARDS, R.C.: Multiple cutaneous and subcutaneous lesions
   occurring simultaneously with hereditary polyposis and osteomatosis. Am.J.hum.
   Genet. 5: 139–147 (1953).

9 GIFFORD, R.D.; GOREE, J., and JIMINEZ, J.P.: Tumor bulge into sphenoid sinus.
   Roentgen sign of parasellar meningioma. Am.J.Roentg. 112: 324–328 (1971).

10 GORLIN, R.J.; MESKIN, L.H., and BRODY, R.: Odontogenic tumors in man and ani-
   mals. Ann.N.Y.Acad.Sci. 108: 722 (1963).

11 HULTH, A. and OLERUD, S.: The reaction of bone to experimental cancer. Acta orthop.
   scand. 36: 230–240 (1965).

12 KENDALL, B.: Invasion of facial bone by basal meningioma. Br.J.Radiol. 46: 237–244
   (1973).

13 KIRKWOOD, J.R.; MARGOLIS, M.T., and NEWTON, T.H.: Prostatic metastasis to base
   of skull simulating meningioma en plaque. Am.J.Roentg. 112: 774–778 (1971).

14 LEEDS, N. and SEAMAN, W.B.: Fibrous dysplasia of skull and its differential diagnosis.
   Radiology 78: 570–582 (1962).

15 LICHTENSTEIN, L. and JAFFE, H.L.: Fibrous dysplasia of bone. Archs Path. 33: 777–816
   (1942).

16 MITCHELL, R.G. and MacLEOD, W.: Leontiasis ossea due to Albers-Schönberg
   disease. Br.J.Radiol. 25: 442–445 (1952).

17a NOYEK, A.M.; HOLGATE, R.C.; WORTZMAN, G.; STEINHARDT, M.I.; SIMOR, I.S.;
    MISKIN, M., and GREYSON, M.D.: Sophisticated radiology in otolaryngology. I. Di-
    agnostic imaging. Roentgenographic (X-ray) modalities. J.Otolar. 6: suppl.3,
    pp.73–94 (1977).

Fig. 27. Metastatic carcinoma of prostate, to frontal sinus and skull. A Caldwell view demonstrates diffuse osteoblastic increase involving almost the entire cranial vault and related structures such as the greater wing of sphenoid of the left (black arrow). The increase in bone thickness and density is characteristic of metastatic prostate cancer in bone. An airfluid level is noted in the left frontal sinus (white arrow), presumably due to hemorrhagic effusion. An old left frontal craniotomy vault defect is noted as well. From ZIZMOR and NOYEK [33].

17b NOYEK, A.M.; ZIZMOR, J., and WORTZMAN, G.: Osteoma of the maxillary sinus – its occurrence following surgery. Can.J.Otol. *3:* 901 (1974).

18 POTTER, G.D.: Sclerosis of base of skull as manifestation of nasopharyngeal carcinoma. J.Radiol. *94:* 35–38 (1970).

19 REED, R.J.: Fibrous dysplasia of bone: a review of 25 cases. Archs Path. *75:* 480–495 (1965).

20 SCHAERER, J.P. and WHITNEY, R.L.: Prostatic metastasis simulating intracranial meningioma. J.Neurosurg. *10:* 546–549 (1973).

21 SCHACTER, I.B.; WORTZMAN, G., and NOYEK, A.M.: The clinical and radiologic diagnosis of cartilaginous tumours of the base of the skull. Can.J.Otol. *2:* 364–377 (1975).

22 SHAPIRO, H. and JANZEN, A.H.: Osteoblastic metastasis to floor of skull simulating meningioma en plaque. Am.J.Roentg. *81:* 964–966 (1959).

23 TSAI, F.Y.; LISELLA, R.F.; LEE, K.F., and ROACH, J.F.: Osteosclerosis of base of skull as a manifestation of tumor invasion. Am.J.Roentg. *124:* 256–264 (1975).

24 NOSTRAND, R.W.P. VAN: Pathologic aspects of osseous and fibro-osseous lesions of the maxillary sinus. Otolar.Clins N.Am. *9:* 35–42 (1976).

25 YOUNG, F.W. and PUTNEY, F.J.: Ossifying fibroma of the sinuses. Ann.Otol.Rhinol. Lar. *77:* 425–434 (1968).

26 ZIZMOR, J. and NOYEK, A.M.: Cysts, benign tumors and mal'gnant tumors of the paranasal sinuses. Otolar.Clins N.Am. *6:* 489–508 (1973).

27 ZIZMOR, J. and NOYEK, A.M.: Cysts and benign tumors of the paranasal sinuses. Sem. Roentg. *3:* 172–201 (1968).

28 ZIZMOR, J.; NOYEK, A.M., and CHAPNIK, J.S.: Mucocele of the paranasal sinuses. Can.J.Otol., suppl. 1 (1974).

29 ZIZMOR, J. and NOYEK, A.M.: Radiology of the nose and paranasal sinuses; in PAPARELLA and SHUMRICK Otolaryngology (Saunders, Philadelphia 1973).

30 ZIZMOR, J. and NOYEK, A.M.: Radiology of the nose and paranasal sinuses; in ENGLISH Otolaryngology (Harper & Row, Hagerstown 1973).

31 ZIZMOR, J. and NOYEK, A.M.: Radiologic diagnosis of maxillary sinus disease. Otolar. Clins N.Am. *9:* 93–115 (1976).

32 ZIZMOR, J. and NOYEK, A.M.: Calcifying and osteoblastic tumours of the paranasal sinuses. J.Otolar. *6:* suppl. 3, pp. 22–44 (1977).

33 ZIZMOR, J. and NOYEK, A.M.: An atlas of otolaryngologic radiology (Saunders, Philadelphia 1978).

ARNOLD M.NOYEK, MD, FRCS (C), FACS, 99 Avenue Road, No.207, *Toronto, Ont. M5R 2G5* (Canada)

Adv. Oto-Rhino-Laryng., vol. 24, pp. 143–165 (Karger, Basel 1978)

Thermography of the Neck

A. Chiesa and L. Acciarri

Department of Radiology, University Hospital, Verona

Introduction

Different body regions diffuse the heat according to their superficial temperature; therefore the possibility of detecting the temperature of skin areas by means of some instruments permits one to evaluate the thermometrical differences existing in each body region.

Skin temperature is closely related to the anatomical (vascular) and functional (metabolic) situation of the region: this relation is the background of the different thermal patterns which are represented in the thermograms. Several lesions modify the thermal pattern of the involved areas and, in some instances, those of the surrounding ones; modifications correspond to an increase (hyperthermia) or – more rarely – to a decrease (hypothermia) of the skin temperature.

Medical thermography permits the recording of the heat of the superficial areas by detecting the infrared radiations which are emitted through the skin and which can be represented on a video screen (dynamic telethermography). The aim of thermography is to detect not only superficial but also deep thermic processes which manifest themselves with skin temperature modifications. For this reason thermogram variations can be related to local pathological lesions.

The applications of medical thermography are well known in breast cancer detection [GHYS, 1973], but they are extended to bone tumors [AARTS, 1969], to cutaneous grafts [DONATI, 1975], to peripheral arterial diseases [LOVISATTI et al., 1975], to cerebral vascular lesions [WALLACE, 1969], and to many other fields.

Thermographic investigation depends on two essential conditions: skin surface suitable for irradiating the heat, and thermal differences from one area to another above a certain level (0.2 °C) in order to obtain a thermogram with different temperature areas represented.

The *neck* is an area which is suitable for thermographic investigation as the essential conditions attain in it; that is: (1) surface easily explored by means of thermography; (2) characteristic thermogram; (3) existence of deep structures which give a superficial thermal manifestation (vessels, glands, etc.), and (4) modifications of the thermogram related to several lesions.

Thermographic Anatomy

The normal neck thermogram has not yet been established [CALVET *et al.*, 1973]. Therefore, the possibility of comparing pathological thermograms to a standard one is not yet possible. We tried to define a normal thermogram which takes into account individual variations and which could be suitable for these comparisons. The normal temperature distribution is represented in figure 1 where the main thermal areas of the neck are shown, each of them characterized by temperature values defined according to three different levels (hot, warm, and cool).

The *normal thermogram* has been based on two standard views: (1) lateral oblique with slightly extended head, and (2) frontal, with hyperextended head.

In the lateral view the following areas are identified (fig. 2).

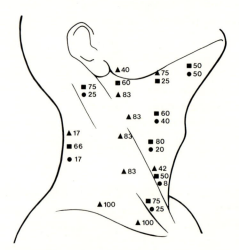

Fig. 1. Normal thermal distribution in the different areas of the neck. Numbers indicate the percentage of occurrence of cool (●), warm (■) and hot (▲) values.

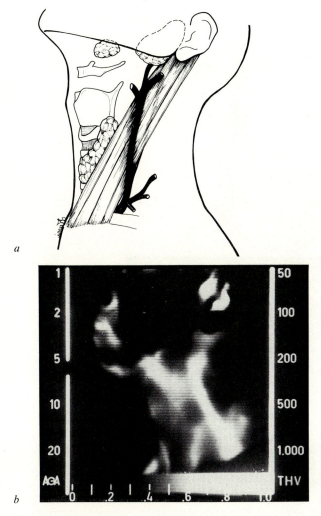

Fig. 2. Lateral view. *a* Anatomic illustration of the regions explored by thermography. *b* Normal thermogram.

Parotid area. The region has a thermographic pattern which is constantly warm or hot because of the superficial situation of the parotid gland and of the vascular structures (external jugular vein and external carotid artery) which pass through the gland. A part of the parotid gland is covered by the masseter muscle and therefore it appears cool; on the other hand this part of the gland does not really belong to the neck but to the facial area.

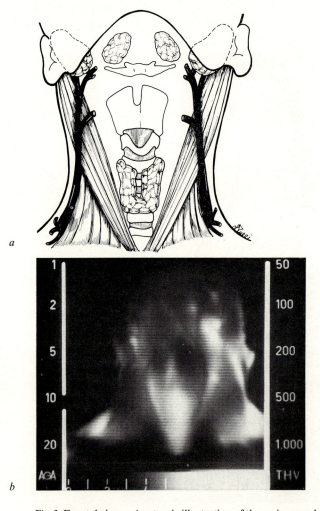

a

b

Fig. 3. Frontal view. *a* Anatomic illustration of the regions explored by thermography. *b* Normal thermogram.

Supra- and subhyoid areas. These two regions are represented on a small surface when investigated on the lateral view. Their thermal characteristics are described in the frontal view.

Sternocleidomastoid area. The correspondence of this region to the sternocleidomastoid muscle explains the extension of warm values. The region is crossed by an hot line directed downwards and posteriorly and which corresponds to the external jugular vein.

Supraclavicular area. It represents the posterior part of the neck, corresponding to scalenus and trapezius muscles. It has almost always warm and uniform values. In its inferior part there is an hot spot which corresponds to vascular structures irradiating from this zone.

Vascular lines. They have very hot values and reach the supraclavicular hyperthermal region coming down from the region of the mandibular angle and surrounding the posterior aspect of the sternocleidomastoid muscle.

The frontal view permits the identification of the following regions (fig. 3).

Suprahyoid area. The normal thermographic pattern of this region is constantly characterized by warm or cool values. Nevertheless, on both sides of the midline just below the jaw in the submaxillary region, an area presenting hot or warm values is constantly recognizable. It could correspond, in its posterior aspect, to the submaxillary gland and, in its anterior aspect, to a branch of the facial artery crossing the platysma and reaching the subcutaneous tissues. Anterior jugular veins which lie on both sides of the midline in the superficial planes do not give a constant thermographically valuable pattern.

Subhyoid area. This region is characterized by warm or cool values whose pattern is not homogeneous, the thermal values progressively increasing from above downwards. The superior third of the region is normally cool (larynx and thyroid cartilage), while the inferior two-thirds are usually warm (thyroid gland).

Sternocleidomastoid area. This region is well examined – in the frontal view – only in the inferior two thirds, its upper part being situated in the lateral aspect of the neck. The vascular line is easily recognizable in this view, too.

Supraclavicular area. A very limited part of this region is recognizable in the frontal view and has always a hyperthermal pattern. This is due to the inferior tract of the external jugular vein and to several small venous branches which are superficial at this point of the area.

Parotid area. This region is seldom identified in the frontal view. It appears on upper external zones of the neck when parotid glands are enlarged.

Pathological Findings

The description of the neck thermograms reveals that the differences which normally exist among the neck temperatures are mainly due to anatomical reasons, such as the site and the level of vascular structures. Nevertheless, some differences are due to the functional activity of very particular regions, such as the parotid and thyroid glands.

The lesions of the neck structures may present different thermographic patterns, which are similar to other regions, that is lesions with increased temperature (hyperthermia), lesions with decreased temperature (hypothermia), and lesions with no variations of the temperature (normothermia). The temperature variations may be isolated to a single region of the neck or be widespread to several regions which are contemporarily attained.

The description takes into account the thermal modifications which can be encountered in the different neck regions. For an easier description sternocleidomastoid and supraclavicular areas will be named laterocervical region.

Parotid Region

It is attained by many lesions with some very typical thermographic patterns. The diagnostics of this region sometimes is not easily performed by sialographic and radioisotopic techniques [BRANDS, 1972]. For these reasons the thermographic technique may constitute a valuable tool for improving the diagnostic results in this area.

Inflammatory processes. They are due to infectious diseases such as in parotitis, or to inflammatory lesions which reach the gland by an ascending route (sialodochitis and sialoadenitis). In both cases a hyperthermia characterizes the inflammation and it exceeds the limits of the gland with an extended hot spot (fig. 4). In some cases chronic inflammatory lesions result in a functional death of the parotid gland which appears on the thermogram as a hypothermal area, in spite of existing inflammatory modifications of the parotid ducts (fig. 5).

Collagenous lesions. The participation of salivary glands to several collagenous diseases has been widely investigated and sialographic manifestations are extensively described in the literature. Thermographic manifestations of these diseases in the parotid area are often recognized. The temperature modification may be detected as an increase of thermal values when the gland is still in the early or intermediate inflammatory phases (fig. 6). The late phases of many collagenous diseases conduct towards an atrophic state of the salivary glands and this situation is thermographically detected as an extended cool pattern of the whole parotid area (fig. 7).

For these reasons it should be possible to check by thermography the progression of the collagenous involvement in salivary glands related to

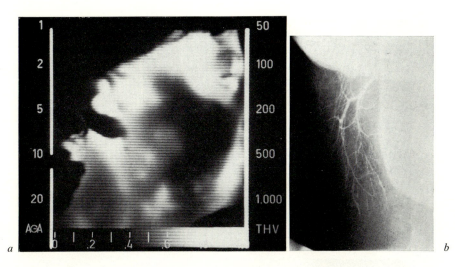

Fig. 4. Acute parotitis. *a* Lateral thermogram showing a hyperthermal area extended to the right preauricolar, retromandibular and submandibular regions. *b* A slight hyperplasia of the parotid gland is revealed on the sialographic examination.

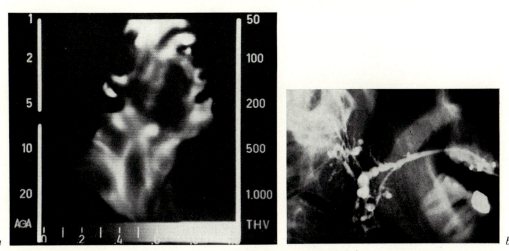

Fig. 5. Chronic parotitis. *a* Lateral thermogram showing the unusual hypothermia extended to the parotid region and to the mandibular angle. *b* Sialographic pattern denoting a typical involvement of the main ducts.

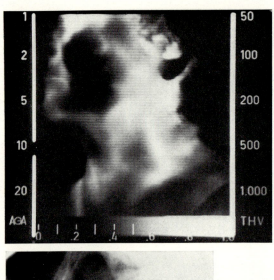

a

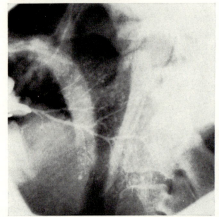

b

Fig.6. Sclerodermia. *a* Lateral thermogram showing a diffuse hyperthermia extended to the parotid and to the submaxillary regions. *b* Sialographic pattern denoting a typical inflammatory phase with several, small, rounded opacities (sialectases).

different temperature values encountered in the corresponding regions (parotid and submaxillary areas).

Benign masses. They are difficult to be clinically differentiated from the mixed tumors which are among the most common masses of the region. Sometimes sialography shows the parotid gland integrity, but in some instances the intraglandular ducts are displaced as in mixed tumors and sialography is not consistent. Benign masses are characterized by warm normal

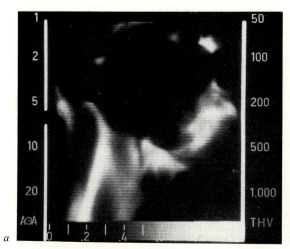
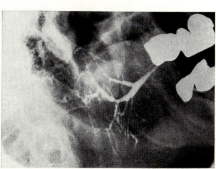

a   *b*

Fig. 7. Sjögren disease. *a* Lateral thermogram showing the extension of the hypothermia to the parotid and to the submaxillary regions. *b* Sialographic appearance of the
right parotid gland in the same subject: ducts are very poor and short.

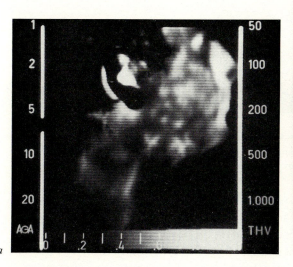
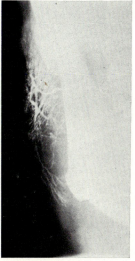

a   *b*

Fig. 8. Salivary cyst. *a* The lateral thermogram shows a thermal pattern within the
normal limits in spite of some distribution irregularities. *b* The sialographic examination
shows a small rounded defect in the inferior half of the gland (cyst).

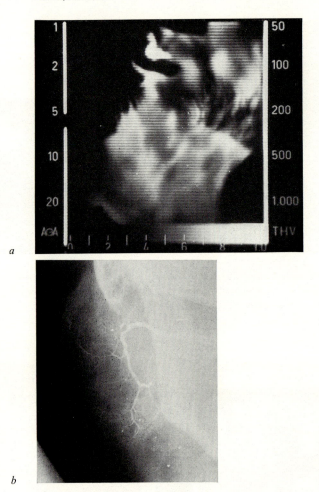

Fig. 9. Parotid lipomatosis. *a* On the lateral thermogram, a hypothermal area covers the parotid and mandibular angle regions. *b* Sialographic examination: the parotid gland presents the ducts displaced by large, lipomatous masses.

thermographic values as in the salivary cysts (fig. 8) or by cool values as in the lypomatous disease of the gland (fig. 9).

A case of an enormous dysontogenetic cyst with necrotic phenomena, situated at the mandibular angle and displacing outwards the inferior aspect of the parotid gland, appeared very cool, probably due to the avascular mass with necrosis (fig. 10).

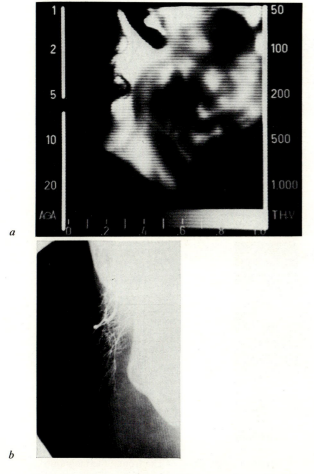

a

b

Fig. 10. Dysontogenetic cyst. *a* On the lateral thermogram, a large hypothermal area is localized on the mandibular angle, just below the inferior aspect of the parotid area. *b* Sialographic appearance of the displaced parotid gland which is not involved by the cyst.

Mixed or malignant masses. The description of mixed and malignant tumors together derives from the fact that they are all characterized by hyperthermal values on the thermogram. Nevertheless the hyperthermal modification due to a mixed tumor (fig. 11) is generally less noticeable and more limited than that of other malignancies, where the spread of the hot temperature outside the parotid region signifies the extensive involvement of the surrounding structures (fig. 12). This latter thermographical pattern

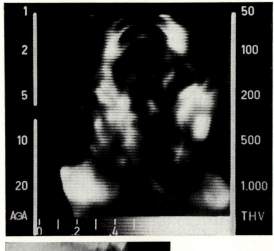

a

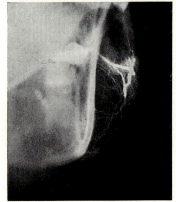

b

Fig. 11. Mixed tumor of the left parotid gland. *a* The frontal thermogram shows a hyperthermal area at the inferior pole of the parotid region. *b* Sialographic examination: the ducts are regularly displaced by the tumor.

may be also encountered when primary tumors situated outside the parotid region spread into it during their growth (fig. 13).

Suprahyoid Region

The thermographic importance of this region is due to the submaxillary glands contained, the lesions of which may give characteristic temperature modifications. Moreover, the superficial projection of these glands being very limited, regional abnormalities can be easily detected.

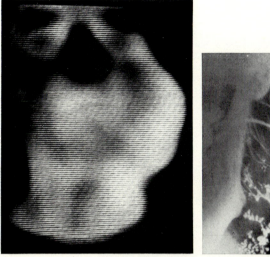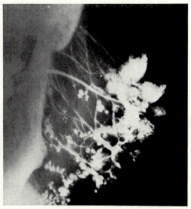

a   b

Fig. 12. Reticulum cell sarcoma of the left parotid gland. *a* The frontal thermogram shows an extended hyperthermal area corresponding to the mass involving the parotid structures. *b* Sialographic examination: enlarged parotid gland with distorted ducts and irregular contrast medium opacities.

Lithiasis. The lesion is the most common disease affecting the submaxillary glands. In general it does not give important modifications on the thermogram: temperature values may be in the range or below the normal ones (fig. 14).

Inflammatory lesions. Consistent temperature modifications are encountered when inflammatory lesions are superimposed to a lithiasis. In these cases the thermographic pattern is analogous to the modification of sialoadenitis where the hot values characterize the disease (fig. 15). In some instances the inflammatory lesion does not originate from the submaxillary gland. The whole suprahyoid region may be invaded by a very hot area with extension to the adjacent subhyoid region when phlegmon infections are localized to the mouth floor (fig. 16).

Subhyoid Region

The importance of this region in thermography is related to thyroid diseases [PLANIOL *et al.*, 1971]. Nevertheless, some other abnormalities may present a thermographic modification of this region.

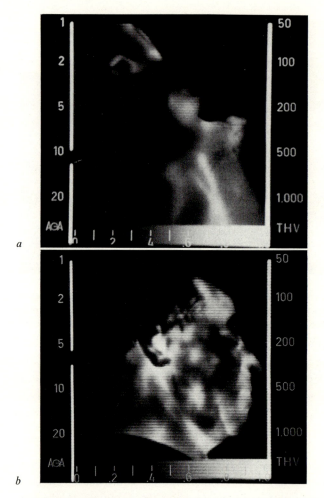

Fig.13. a Recurrence of a skin tumor. The left parotid area is hyperthermal in the preauricular zone where the primary malignancy was localized. *b* External auditory meatus tumor. The hyperthermal pattern is localized to the external meatus and to the parotid/submaxillary areas.

Larynx and pharynx tumors. The hyperthermal modification which laryngeal and pharyngeal malignancies may present, is not easily conducible to a schematic representation. When hyperthermia is evident it has generally a very extended pattern and it does not correspond closely to the anatomic lesions. This may be due to the relatively deep structures involved in these tumors (fig. 17). Nevertheless the identification of the most affected side is

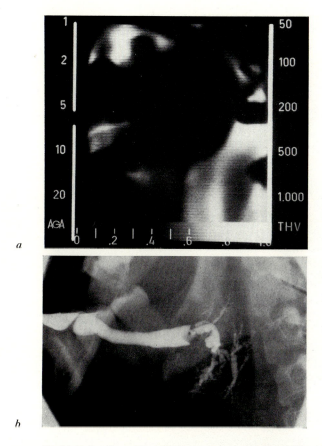

Fig. 14. Left submaxillary lithiasis. *a* Lateral thermogram showing cool temperature values in the submaxillary area. *b* Sialographic evidence of the lithiasis with the filling defect in the duct.

possible and this fact permits one to study adequately the treatment planning: the importance of this study is evident due to the frequent coexistence of metastatic nodes.

Laterocervical Region

The region comprises the two anatomical areas formerly described as sternocleidomastoid and supraclavicular areas. The opportunity of describing

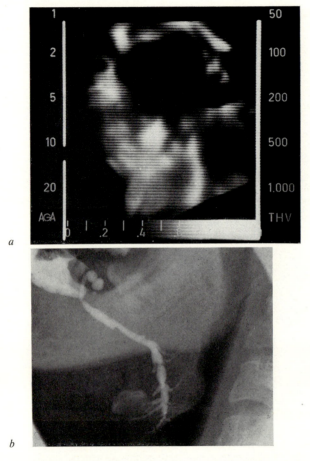

Fig. 15. Right submaxillary sialoadenitis. *a* The lateral thermogram reveals a marked hyperthermia in the submaxillary gland area. *b* Sialography denotes a diffuse sialodochitis with poor intraglandular ducts.

them together as a single region derives from the distribution of pathological lesions which affect indifferently one or both areas and by the fact that thermal modifications may be widespread in the whole regional surface.

Vascular abnormalities. When increased vascularity occurs, the best situation for thermographic modifications is realized. Vascular changes in the arterovenous fistulas of the neck (fig. 18) are easily detected by thermography, appearing as an hot spot in the area of the more superficial vascular involve-

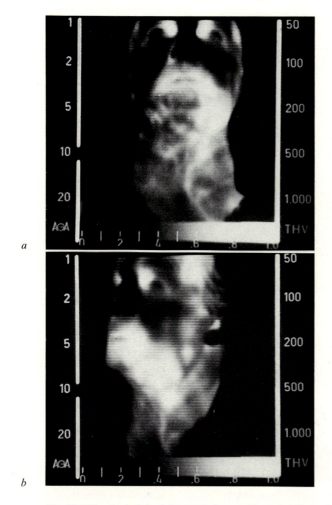

Fig. 16. Phlegmon of the left mouth floor. *a* Frontal. *b* Lateral thermograms showing the very extended hyperthermal area affecting the supra- and subhyoid regions.

ment. Sometimes the vascular involvement is clinically evident as a well limited, palpable, pulsating mass in the laterocervical region, with an extended hyperthermia on the thermogram. In the case of figure 19, the intervention demonstrated the presence of chemodectoma originating from the carotid bifurcation and greatly extended upwards.

Vascular modifications constantly occur when a radiation therapy is performed. The thermographic detection of these changes in the laterocervical

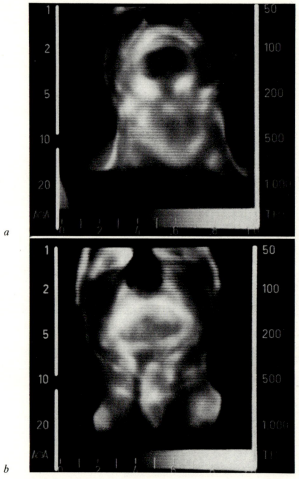

Fig. 17. a Laryngeal cancer. Thermogram in frontal view showing a hyperthermal area situated in the midline of the subhyoid region. *b* Cancer of the left piriform sinus. Thermogram in frontal view, showing the left side of the subhyoid region with an extended hyperthermal zone.

area is a good method for evaluating the tissue response to the absorbed doses. WHITE *et al.* [1975] propose the thermographic evaluation of the temperature changes in the laterocervical area following preoperative radiotherapy, as a tool for proposing the most opportune time in head and neck cancer surgery.

Lymphatic node lesions. The involvement of lymphatic nodes characterizes a great deal of laterocervical pathological conditions. The primary

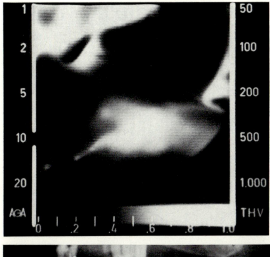

a

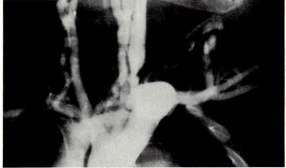

b

Fig. 18. Arterovenous fistulas of the neck in a child. *a* Lateral thermogram with hyperextended head. The supraclavicular area is highly hyperthermal. *b* Aortic arch angiography.
Large fistulas are recognized at the left carotid artery and left subclavian artery origin;
at the supraclavicular region is another fistulous area.

lymphomatous lymph node involvement do not belong to the ORL field of
interest. The detection and localization of the metastatic secondary nodes is
much more important from the laryngological point of view. Laryngeal
cancer may be accompanied by metastatic nodes in the neck region. On the
other hand, recurrences of operated laryngeal cancers are almost exclusively
localized to these regions. Figure 20 shows the not homogeneous, hyperthermal pattern of a patient operated by laryngectomy, having an extended
recurrence affecting the laterocervical lymphatic nodes. In many other cases
it was possible to detect the invasion of lymphatic nodes by carcinomatous
metastasis originating from the parotid, the larynx or the pharynx.

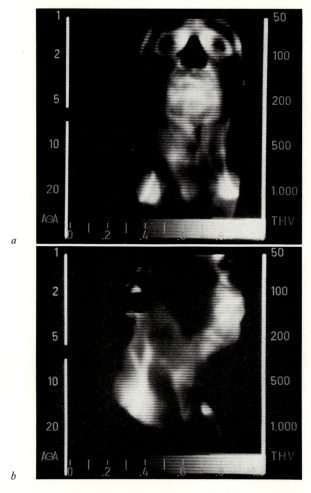

Fig. 19. Chemodectoma of the right carotid bifurcation. *a* Frontal. *b* Lateral thermograms showing an extended hyperthermal area situated outside the carotid axis, just forward the sternocleidomastoid muscle.

Conclusions

The role of thermography in the neck lesions is not yet sufficiently defined. Almost all lesions affecting the neck structures give a thermographic evidence of their existence.

The thermographic modifications are mainly hyperthermal, but hypothermal patterns are not unusual. Moreover thermal characteristics are often

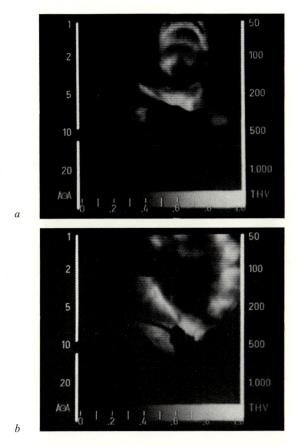

Fig. 20. Operated larynx cancer. *a* Frontal. *b* Lateral thermograms showing an extended hyperthermal area involving both the laterocervical lymphatic chains and the supra- sub-hyoid regions.

identical in many diseases. Hyperthermia, for example, is evident in inflammatory lesions and in malignancies.

To distinguish these two kinds of hyperthermia a quantitative evaluation is necessary.

The thermal gradient (Δ t) between two areas' temperature, is the quantitative measure which thermography makes possible (table I). The thermal gradient permits one to compare the temperature differences between adjacent areas and, when possible, between symmetric regions. The great number of variations in the thermographic neck pattern practically requires that any temperature modification is quantitatively evaluated by thermal gradient.

Table I. Average thermic gradient existing between sternocleidomastoid area and other head and neck regions.

	Δt
Cheek	−1.50
Suprahyoid	−1.00
Subhyoid (upper half), and supraclavicular (upper half)	−0.50
Sternocleidomastoid	=
Subhyoid (inferior half) and parotid	+0.50
Submaxillary and supraclavicular (inferior half)	+1.00
Vascular lines	+1.50

With this kind of evaluation, the primary tumor hyperthermia, for example, results much higher ($\Delta t = 3\,°C$) than that of the secondary lymphatic nodes involvement ($\Delta t = 1.5\,°C$). In addition, thermography is a valuable method for evaluating the evolution of many diseases. The method permits one to check the vascular or functional modification of some regions, either in chronic conditions as in collagenous and tumoral lesions, or in acute manifestations as in inflammatory diseases.

The role of thermography as a bloodless method for detecting or checking many neck lesions should be further clarified. It must be stressed that thermography alone is not sufficient for an exact definition of the nature of the lesions. Thermography should be linked to other diagnostic examinations such as sialography, radioisotopic studies, tomography etc. In this role it has certainly good chances for improving its value.

Summary

The thermographic investigation of the neck is described. The normal thermographic pattern of different neck areas is tabulated according to lateral oblique and frontal views. Hot, warm and cool values define different areas, producing the characteristic neck thermogram. Lesions of the neck modify the normal thermogram, and they are differentiated according to the site of origin. Parotid, suprahyoid, subhyoid, and laterocervical regions are described together with their pathological modifications.

The validity of thermography in neck lesions seems to be consistent with these points:

Salivary gland lesions are easily recognizable because of the superficial position of these structures. Moreover the temperature modifications have almost always a good concordance with the lesion nature.

Pharynx and larynx lesions are scarcely detectable because the involvement of these structures must be greatly extended before the temperature modification reaches the superficial planes.

Lymphatic node lesions do not present characteristic features permitting an accurate diagnosis of their localization in the neck, except for the hyperthermal values which characterize the carcinomatous origin.

Vascular abnormalities have a good chance to be detected because of the high increase of temperature they cause.

References

AARTS, N.J.M.: Thermography in malignant and inflammatory diseases of the bones; in Medical thermography. Biblthca radiol., No. 5, pp. 182–190 (Karger, Basel 1969).

BRANDS, T.: Diagnose und Klinik der Erkrankungen der grossen Kopfspeicheldrüsen (Urban & Schwarzenberg, München 1972).

CALVET, J.; TOROSSIAN, F., et al.: Apport de la téléthermographie dynamique en cancérologie cervico-faciale. Méditer. méd. 2: 38–40 (1973).

DONATI, L.: Téléthermographie en chirurgie plastique. Actes 9e Congr. Radiol. Cult. Lat. J. Radiol. Electrol. 56: suppl. 1, p. 55 (1975).

GHYS, R.: Thermographie médicale, pp. 109–170 (Maloine, Paris 1973).

LOVISATTI, L.; MORA, L., and PISTOLESI, G.F.: Thermographic patterns of lower limb arterial diseases; in Thermography. Biblthca radiol., No. 6. pp. 107–114 (Karger, Basel 1975).

PLANIOL, T.; GARNIER, G. et POURCELOT, L.: L'association de la thermographie et de l'échographie bidimensionnelle à la scintigraphie dans l'étude des nodules froids thyroïdiens. Ann. Radiol. 14: 695–708 (1971).

WALLACE, J.D.: A thermographic indication of carotid insufficiency; in Medical thermography. Biblthca radiol., No. 5, pp. 153–159 (Karger, Basel 1969).

WHITE, R.L.; EL-MAHDI, A.M.; RAMIREZ, H.L.; TEATES, C.D., and CONSTABLE, W.C.: Thermographic changes following preoperative radiotherapy in head and neck cancer. Radiology 117: 469–471 (1975).

Dr. A. CHIESA, Department of Radiology, University Hospital, *I-37100 Verona* (Italy)

Adv. Oto-Rhino-Laryng., vol. 24, pp. 166–169 (Karger, Basel 1978)

Radiological and Pathological Findings of Esthesioneuroblastoma

K. J. Momose, A. L. Weber and M. L. Goodman

Department of Radiology, Massachusetts Eye and Ear Infirmary,
and Massachusetts General Hospital, Boston, Mass.

Olfactory esthesioneuroblastoma is a rare but recognized tumor with definite clinical, radiological, and pathological findings [1, 2]. A total of 25 patients with this tumor were studied over a period of 25 years at the Massachusetts Eye and Ear Infirmary. The tumor is thought to arise from the neurosensory receptor cells of the olfactory mucosa. It is a friable, vascular tumor which usually arises in the nasal fossa. The tumor consists of epithelial as well as neural elements. The predominant 'lymphoid' cells are called esthesioneurocytes which tend to cluster together to form rosettes or pseudorosettes. The diagnosis of this tumor is occasionally difficult to make due to the multiplicity of the cellular pattern. The tumor can be misdiagnosed as anaplastic carcinoma, transitional cell carcinoma, or lymphosarcoma.

In our series there were 14 female and 11 male cases. The age range was from 3 to 76 years, with a peak range between 11–21 and 31–40 years. The tumor is usually slow-growing as it originates in and extends from the superolateral portion of the nasal cavity into the contiguous ethmoid sinuses. The other sinuses are sometimes involved directly or indirectly. Due to the position of this tumor, the patient often complains of nasal obstruction, epistaxis, or sinusitis. When this tumor is incompletely removed it has a tendency to recur and spread. It can invade the retrobulbar space of the orbit or extend into the anterior or middle cranial fossa. 6% of the tumor can go to distant metastasis. Our cases were grouped and analyzed under three categories: (1) tumor confined to the nasal fossa (7 cases), (2) tumor confined to the nasal fossa and the contiguous paranasal sinuses (5 cases), (3) tumor extending beyond the paranasal sinuses into the retrobulbar space and/or intracranially (13 cases). The common radiological findings were as follows: (1) all had some degree of opacification of one or more of the paranasal sinuses due to direct

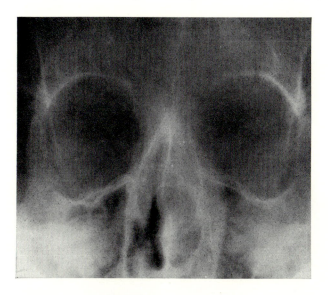

Fig. 1. Tumor in the left nasal cavity extending into the ethmoid sinuses with destruction of the medial orbital wall.

tumor invasion or related to occlusion of the opening into the paranasal sinuses, (2) 12 cases had a mass in the nasal fossa or in the paranasal sinuses, (3) almost all cases show bony destruction of the lateral wall of the nasal fossa or the contiguous paranasal sinus, (4) 7 cases were studied by angiography and the tumor was vascular in 3, slightly vascular in 1, and avascular in 2. Two cases demonstrated an avascular as well as a vascular component. Computed tomography was used to study 4 advanced cases to rule out invasion in the retrobulbar space or intracranially. The tumor extends into the retrobulbar space in 3 and intracranially in 3.

Although this tumor is radiosensitive it tends to recur frequently unless completely eradicated. Of the 17 patients who were followed in our series, 15 (76%) were alive without disease following radical surgery, radiation, or a combination of the two methods. Uncontrolled primary lesions with or without metastases accounted for all the therapeutic failures. Even with intracranial extension of this tumor, people have survived from 2 to 5 years with surgery or radiotherapy. In recent years more patients have survived due to well-planned surgical and radiotherapeutic procedures, resulting from better demonstration of the tumor by new diagnostic techniques.

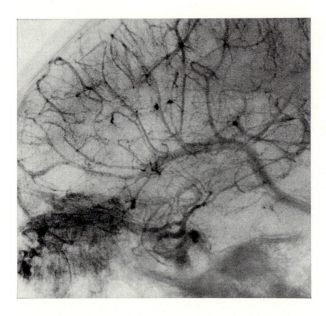

Fig. 2. Carotid angiogram reveals tumor vascularity with extension through the cribiform plate into the anterior cranial fossa.

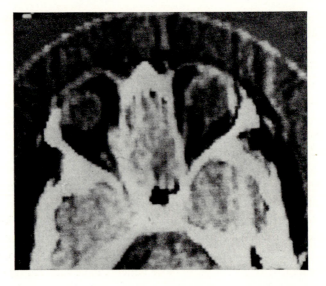

Fig. 3. Computerized axial tomogram showing tumor in the nasal cavity and ethmoids with extension into the left retroorbital space.

Case Report

A 60-year-old male complained of nasal obstruction without symptoms relating to the central nervous system. A biopsy of a polyp protruding from the nasal fossa on the left side proved to be an esthesioneuroblastoma. The paranasal sinus films showed complete opacification of the nasal fossa and the ethmoid sinus on the left side (fig. 1). A left carotid angiogram (fig. 2) demonstrated a large vascular tumor in the left ethmoid sinus with extension into the anterior and middle cranial fossa. A CT scan (fig. 3) showed a soft tissue mass in the nasal fossa and the ethmoid sinus with some extension of the tumor through the medial wall of the left retrobulbar space.

Due to the size of this tumor with extension intracranially, it was decided to treat this patient with radiotherapy rather than radical surgery.

References

1   KADISH, S.; GOODMAN, M., and WANG, C.C.: Olfactory neuroblastoma, a clinical analysis of 17 cases. Cancer 37: 1571–1576 (1976).
2   HUTTER, R.; LEWIS, J.S.; FOOTE, F.W., jr., and TOLLEFSEN, H.R.: Esthesioneuroblastoma, a clinical and pathological study. Am.J.Surg. 106: 748–752 (1963).

Dr. A.L.WEBER, Massachusetts Eye and Ear Infirmary, Department of Radiology, Massachusetts General Hospital, Boston, MA 02114 (USA)

Adv. Oto-Rhino-Laryng., vol. 24, pp. 170–176 (Karger, Basel 1978)

Tracheal Tumors:
Radiological, Clinical and Pathological Evaluation

A. L. WEBER and H. C. GRILLO

Department of Radiology, Massachusetts Eye and Ear Infirmary,
and Department of Surgery, Massachusetts General Hospital,
Harvard Medical School, Boston, Mass.

Primary tumors of the trachea are rare lesions as opposed to tumors of the larynx and lung, which are 75 and 180 times more frequent [5]. The majority of lesions encountered in the pediatric age group are benign (90%) while the majority of the tumors in the adult are malignant [1,3]. The incidence of tracheal carcinomas is less than 0.1% in patients dying of cancer [5,9]. Tracheal tumors are classified into: (1) benign tumors, (2) primary malignant tumors of the trachea, (3) primary malignant tumors involving the trachea and larynx, (4) primary malignant tumors of the lower trachea extending into the bronchi, and (5) malignant tumors with secondary tracheal involvement most often originating from lung, esophagus, and thyroid. The majority of primary tracheal tumors are squamous cell carcinomas followed by adenoid cystic carcinomas [4,5]. The peak incidence of carcinoma of the trachea is between 50 and 60 years of age while the incidence of adenoid cystic carcinoma is about 10 years earlier. Most common benign tumors encountered in the trachea in the pediatric age group are squamous cell papilloma, hemangioma and fibroma [3]. Malignant tumors of the trachea may be preceded or followed with an interval of several years by other tumors of the respiratory tract and digestive tract [4]. Among 27 primary carcinomas of the trachea in our series, there were 5 patients with a second primary tumor, 3 in the larynx and 2 in the lung.

Clinical Manifestations [4, 5, 7, 9]

Interpretation of the clinical symptoms in the diagnosis is difficult because of the vague localizing signs, the usual negative chest X-ray, and the healthy appearance of the patient. The symptoms are often insidious in onset and often occur in the later stages of the disease. At least 75% or more of the tracheal lumen needs to be obstructed before there are any localizing symptoms. The average duration of symptoms from onset to diagnosis is about 12–15 months in malignant lesions [5], and often a much longer interval in benign lesions. The symptoms encountered in our group of patients with primary benign and malignant tumors were in order of frequency, dyspnea, hemoptysis, cough, wheezing, dysphagia, change in voice and/or hoarseness, stridor, and pneumonia. Nine patients were treated for asthma and emphysema, mistakenly in the presence of a tumor within the trachea.

Pathological Features

Benign lesions are intraluminal, often less than 2 cm in diameter and may be broad-based or on a stalk. They do not extend beyond the tracheal wall into the adjacent mediastinal structures. Squamous cell papillomas often have their initial occurrence in the larynx and in a small percentage of cases, they extend by secondary seeding to the trachea, and in rare instances to bronchi and lung. They are polypoid in configuration and often are multiple.

Most malignant lesions are about 2–4 cm in greatest diameter, but lesions as long as 10 cm have been observed. Tracheal carcinomas often occur in the posterior lateral wall, spread intraluminally and sooner or later will penetrate the trachea with invasion of adjacent structures such as paratracheal lymph nodes, esophagus, vascular structures, larynx, and thyroid. In a small percentage of cases, distant metastases to lung, skeleton, liver, kidneys, adrenals, abdominal lymph nodes, brain, heart, including pericardium have been reported. The squamous cell carcinoma varies from poorly differentiated small cell type to the pearl-forming squamous variety [4]. Adenoid cystic carcinoma is characterized by cords and sheets of fairly uniform small cells and cyst-like structures of various size. The tumor often penetrates the tracheal wall and invades paratracheal tissue [8]. Perineural extension is common in adenoid cystic carcinoma as in other areas of the head and neck region. Five-year survival data is not applicable to adenoid cystic carcinomas since they often recur and may have a prolonged course even in the presence of metastases to distant sites such as the lung. A course of 5–25 years of this tumor is not an uncommon occurrence. The mucus-secreting adenocarcinoma (less common) is often large and bulky with deep penetration into the tracheal wall and adjacent mediastinum. The histology of this tumor is similar to mucus-secreting adenocarcinoma of the lung.

Table I. Radiologic findings

---

1 Polypoid mass
   Benign: sharply defined, often less than 2 cm in size; calcification demonstrated
      in cartilaginous tumor
   Malignant: irregular margin, more broadbased, often greater than 2 cm
2 Irregular Longitudinal intraluminal mass
   A With variable-sized extraluminal component
   B Average length 2–4 cm (range up to 10 cm)
3 Narrowing of the tracheal lumen with a variable-sized mass
4 Indentation or invasion of esophagus, superior vena cava, main bronchi
5 Air trapping, pneumonia, atelectasis if bronchi are involved

---

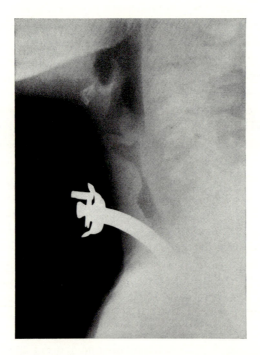

Fig. 1. Fibroma of the trachea. 11-year-old male treated for asthma. Over a period of several years developed progressive dyspnea and stridor. There is a sharply defined homogeneous hemispherical shaped density arising from the anterior wall of the upper trachea and extending into the infraglottic portion of the larynx. Note metallic tracheostomy tube inserted for severe airway obstruction.

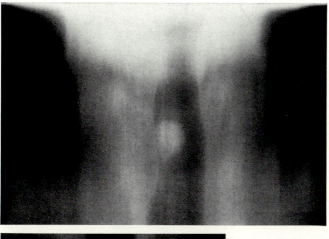

2

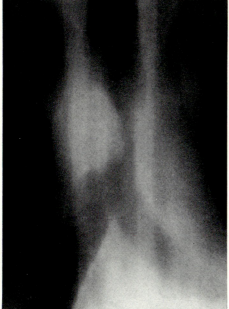

3

Fig. 2. Spindle cell sarcoma of the upper trachea. 15-year-old girl with a history of cough, dyspnea and stridor. Note sharply defined polypoid density arising from the right wall of the trachea.

Fig. 3. Squamous cell carcinoma of the lower third of the trachea. 51-year-old male patient with history of dyspnea and hemoptysis. There is a slightly irregular hemispherical shaped lesion arising from the right wall of the lower third of the trachea above the bifurcation. Note slight thickening and bulging of right tracheal wall suggesting penetration to the mediastinal structures.

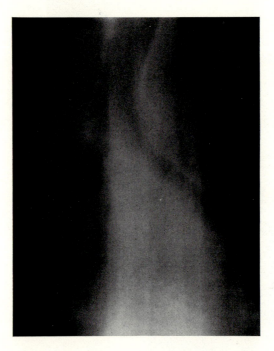

Fig. 4. Squamous cell carcinoma of the lower trachea extending into the main bronchi. 56-year-old male with cough and shortness of breath. There is invasion of the left main stem bronchus by an irregular tumor mass. There is also tumor in the lower third of the trachea which is not clearly defined on this print.

Radiographic Findings [2, 6]

The radiologic modalities applied in the evaluation of tracheal lesions are: (1) preliminary chest film with oblique tracheal views, (2) AP over-penetrated high kV view of the trachea, (3) AP, lateral and oblique linear laminagraphy of the trachea, and (4) fluoroscopy of the trachea and larynx with additional spot films and opacification of the esophagus with barium.

The most important radiological features are outlined in table I. Benign lesions are sharply defined and homogeneous and if calcium is demonstrated a cartilaginous tumor should be considered. Some malignant lesions have a sharply defined polypoid appearance and can simulate benign lesions parti-cularly if they are sarcomatous (fig. 1). Most malignant lesions are flat, irreg-ular, and extend over a variable length along the tracheal wall (fig. 2). In figure 3, the lumen of the trachea is compromised to a variable degree. A

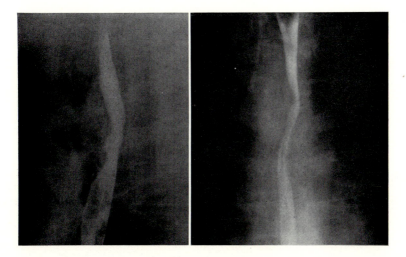

Fig. 5. Adenoid cystic carcinoma of the midtrachea with indentation and displacement of esophagus. 35-year-old male with history of dyspnea and hemoptysis. Oval-shaped mass arising from posterior wall of trachea with extraluminal extension and indentation of the esophagus anteriorly and on the right.

large extraluminal component causing mediastinal widening may be observed on the chest film or by laminagraphy. If the tumor is in the lower portion of the trachea, secondary involvement of the bronchi may occur. In some of these cases, air trapping, atelectasis, and/or pneumonia are demonstrated in the respective lung (fig. 4). The extraluminal tumor component may invade or displace the esophagus as best demonstrated with barium in the esophagus and overhead or oblique spot films in different degrees of rotation. In figure 5, partial or total obstruction of the superior vena cava secondary to invasion by tumor is demonstrated by angiography. If the tumor is in the upper portion of the trachea, simultaneous invasion of the larynx with infraglottic narrowing may occur.

References

1   CALDAROLA, V. T.; HARRISON, E. G., jr.; CLAGETT, O. T., and SCHMIDT, H. W.: Benign tumors and tumorlike conditions of the trachea and bronchi. Ann. Otol. *73:* 1042–1061 (1974).
2   FLEMING, R. J.; MEDINA, J., and SEAMAN, W. B.: Roentgenographic aspects of tracheal tumors. Radiology *79:* 628–636 (1962).

3   Gilbert, J.G.; Mazzarella, L.A., and Feit, L.J.: Primary tracheal tumors in the
     infant and adult. Archs Otolar. *58:* 1–9 (1953).
4   Hajdu, S.I.; Huvos, A.G.; Goodner, J.T.; Foote, F.W., jr., and Beattie, E.J., jr.:
     Carcinoma of the trachea. Clinicopathologic study of 41 cases. Cancer *25:* 1448–1456
     (1970).
5   Houston, H.E.; Payne, W.S.; Harrison, E.G., jr., and Olsen, A.M.: Primary
     cancers of the trachea. Archs Surg. *99:* 132–140 (1969).
6   Janower, M.L.; Grillo, H.C.; Macmillan, A.S., jr., and James, A.E., jr.: The
     radiological appearance of carcinoma of the trachea. Radiology *96:* 39–43 (1970).
7   Moersch, H.J.; Clagett, O.T., and Eliss, F.H.: Tumors of the trachea, Med. Clin.
     N. Am. *38:* 1091–1096 (1954).
8   Pearson, F.G.; Thompson, D.W.; Weissberg, D.; Simpson, W.J.K., and Kergin,
     F.G.: Adenoid cystic carcinoma of the trachea. Ann. thorac. Surg. *18:* 16–29 (1974).
9   Ranke, E.J.; Presley, S.S., and Holinger, P.H.: Tracheogenic carcinoma. J. Am.
     med. Ass. *182:* 121–124 (1962).
10   Smith, L.C.; Lane, N., and Rankow, R.M.: Cylindroma (adenoid cystic carcinoma).
     A report of fifty-eight cases. Am. J. Surg. *110:* 519 (1965).

Dr. A.L. Weber, Massachusetts Eye and Ear Infirmary, Department of Radiology, Massachusetts General Hospital, *Boston, MA 02114* (USA)

Adv. Oto-Rhino-Laryng., vol. 24, pp. 177–196 (Karger, Basel 1978)

A Comparison of Bone Scintigraphy and Tomography in Diseases of Paranasal Sinus and of the Base of the Skull

K. W. Frey, M. Hueber, R. Rohloff, U. Büll and R. Neef

Clinic and Polyclinic of Radiology (Prof. J. Lissner), University of Munich, Munich

Bone-seeking radiopharmaceuticals are currently used to diagnose malignant and benign bone tumors as well as inflammatory and systemic bone diseases. Bone scans obtained with rectilinear scanner, gamma-camera or whole body scanner are widely applied as a screening method to detect metastases, multiple inflammatory bone lesions and bone lesions in morbus Paget and hyperparathyroidism. Scintigraphy is also a valuable tool in early diagnosis, because some bone lesions such as metastases and hematogeneous osteomyelitis are positive on scans earlier than on radiographs [4, 5] (fig. 10). Scans of primary malignant bone tumors and bone metastases show the extent of the lesion, support the operation planning and help to determine the exact field size in radiotherapy. Pure lytic lesions without bone reaction may show a normal scan, but an abnormal radiograph for example in multiple myeloma with multiple punched-out defects, in some osteolytic metastases and in benign bone tumors without a tendency to grow and without an increased bone metabolism. Therefore imaging and tomography are two contributory methods. In any case, a positive scan is supplemented by radiographic examination for better details (fig. 2, 3).

In radiograms with similar bone changes scans make a differential diagnosis possible to discern bone lesions with normal and increased mineral metabolism. So Paget's vertebra always shows an increased radionuclide uptake in contrast to the hemangioma vertebra and the so-called hypertrophic atrophy of the vertebra in osteoporosis. Also an acute spondylitis has an intensively increased tracer accumulation in contrast to spondylosis and vertebral epiphysitis with Schmorl's nodes.

Methods

^{99m}Tc-labeled radiopharmaceuticals are currently the agents of choice for clinical skeletal images. ^{99m}Tc-pyrophosphate, ^{99m}Tc-polyphosphate and ^{99m}Tc-diphosphonate were employed. The usual dose was between 3 and 10 mCi, and the patients were studied 3–9 h after the injection on a rectilinear scanner. ^{99m}Tc is always available from a molybdenum-tin-technetium generator. Using short-living bone-seeking nuclides as ^{99m}Tc-pyrophosphate ($T\frac{1}{2} = 6$ h, ^{87m}Sr ($T\frac{1}{2} = 2.7$ h) and ^{18}fluorine ($T\frac{1}{2} = 1.9$ h) has the disadvantage that the examination has to be performed very early.

The very short postinjection period is necessary because of the fast physical decay. But that period is not optimal for bone scans, because the nuclide is only absorbed to the surface of the bone but not yet incorporated in the matrix, while still there exists a high soft tissue and blood pool activity. The long-living ^{85}Sr ($T\frac{1}{2} = 64$ days) has the advantage of a more suitable bone/soft tissue ratio 2–7 days after injection of 0.1 mCi.

For practical clinical purposes the advantages of short-living bone-seeking radionuclides are: (1) markedly reduced radiation to the patient (10 mCi ^{99m}Tc-pyrophosphate gives an exposure of approximately 1 rad to the bone while 0.1 mCi ^{85}Sr gives 3–6 rads!), and (2) increased counts per minute, because the radioactivity is 30–100 times higher. Scans of the head and sometimes quantifying profiles consist of anterior views (fig. 1a, b) and lateral views (fig. 1c, d).

Techniques of Tomography

Tomograms were done with the 'Polytome' (Philipps-Massiot) with hypocycloidal blurring in 5-mm cuts in a.-p. and lateral views. The angle is 45°, focal spot 1 mm², distance of the focal plane from the film 145 cm. There is a constant magnification of 1.3.

Fig. 1. Normal activity distribution on anterior (a, b) and lateral (c, d) view. *a, c* Normal activity profile, measured with a slit collimator 2 days after intravenous injection of 0.1 mCi ^{85}Sr in 20 normal individuals. A = Eye, Aw = lateral angle of the eye, Aw li = lateral angle of the left eye, Aw re = lateral angle of the right eye, A li = left eye, A re = right eye, MAO = middle of the line eye/ear, N = nose, O = ear. *b, d* Normal activity distribution after intravenous injection of 5–10 mCi ^{99m}Tc-pyrophosphate in percent at different points. Definition: 100% in anterior scan = point at radix nasi; 100% in lateral scan = point before meatus acusticus externus. Mean values and standard deviation in 20 normal subjects.

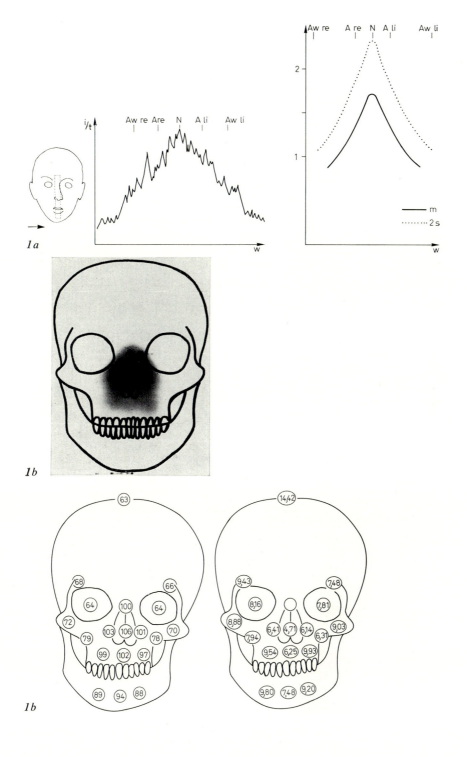

1a

1b

1b

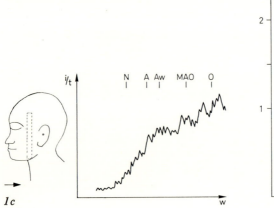
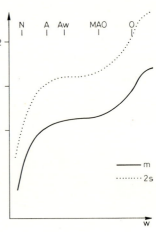

1c

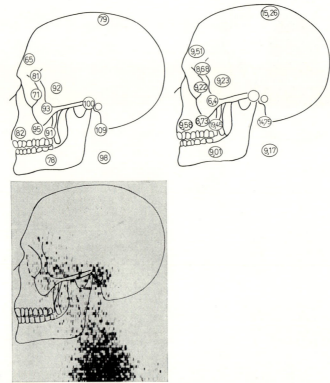

1d

Normal Distribution of Activity in the Scan and Profile

The quantifying profile of ^{85}Sr [5,7,9] shows a marked maximum in the center and parasagittally (fig. 1a) with a radioactivity ratio to both heels of 1.71 ± 30 (2 σ, gained from 15 healthy adults) [9] and a marked slope to the maxillary sinus with an activity ratio of only 1.02 ± 0.20. The ^{99m}Tc-pyrophosphate anterior scan has a sagittally broad radionuclide uptake in projection to the nose with reduced activity laterally over the maxillary sinuses. The lateral part never takes up more than the central part. There is also a symmetric accumulation of right and left side. ^{85}Sr profile (fig. 1c) and ^{99m}Tc-pyrophosphate scan (fig. 1d) have a maximum in projection to the ear in the lateral view. This maximum is more pronounced in the profile than in the scan (fig. 1d). The scintigram shows often more, individually focal increased accumulations over the maxillary sinus. This increased radioactivity is not as intense in healthy individuals as in patients with abnormal radionuclide deposition adjacent to focal sceletal lesions (fig. 2–6).

Facial Bones and Anterior Part of the Skull

Osteoplasia and Osteocondensation

Lesions with Increased Uptake

Expansively growing osteoblastic and ossifying tumors demonstrate a markedly increased uptake of the focus over the facial bones and the fossa anterior. The maximum is shifted ventrally (fig. 2, 3), as in expansively growing osteomas of the frontal sinus, of the ethmoidal sinuses and orbita (fig. 2), osteogenic fibroma [7,8], osteochondromas of the maxillary sinuses [17], osteogenic meningeomas, fibrous dysplasia (fig. 3) and osteogeneous sarcoma. Generally the uptake is homogeneous [7–9]. Extensive lesions have often an inhomogeneous uptake pattern, despite the fact that the tomogram demonstrates a homogeneous density. The site of the maximum uptake corresponds to the most active part of the altered osteogenesis. One may suppose the direction of expansion, as in a fibrous dysplasia, which involved the frontal sinus and the anterior cerebral fossa and showed an intensive maximum over the anterior fossa (fig. 3).

Postoperative scintigraphic follow-ups in longer intervals are used to detect the recurrence of a tumor. A patient with an osteoma of the sphenoid sinus, operated on 2 years earlier, demonstrated a decrease of uptake on the quantitative ^{85}Sr profile over the middle part of the skull base. A recent profile

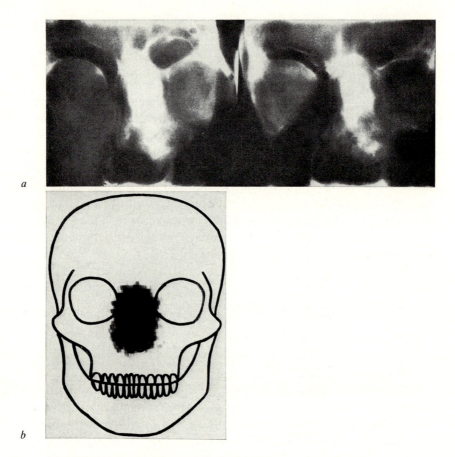

Fig.2. 58-year-old, female. Osteoma of the os ethmoidale with a very intense uptake in the center and well-defined to the surrounding.

and scan showed an increased accumulation over the anterior fossa and frontal sinus. A recurrence of the osteoma was reported ventrally. On surgery the diagnosis was proved.

Lesions with Small or Absent Uptake

In contrast to huge, infiltrative expansive osteomas of the paranasal sinuses with very intensive accretion, four small osteomas with a diameter of 1.0–1.5 cm within the lumen of the frontal sinus and without connection of

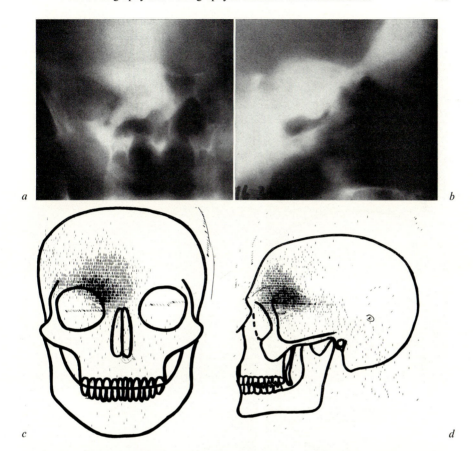

Fig. 3. 23-year-old male. Fibrous dysplasia with very heavy bone condensation of the sphenoid sinus, the anterior cerebral fossa and os frontale. The intensive uptake over the anterior part of the skull base and on the right side corresponds to the increased bone metabolism. But there is only a slightly increased tracer accumulation over the sphenoid sinus.

the anterior or posterior wall of the frontal sinus demonstrated a normal radionuclide deposition pattern. Despite clearly illustrated bone density on the tomogram a 2.5-cm osteoma within the anterior fossa at the crista galli 2 cm behind the posterior wall of the frontal sinus, a 3-cm osteoma of the occipital bone and some not growing up to 5 cm huge osteomas of extremity bones showed negative scans.

The intensity of radioactivity does not only depend on the size but especially on the activity of bone metabolism of these benign bone tumors. A

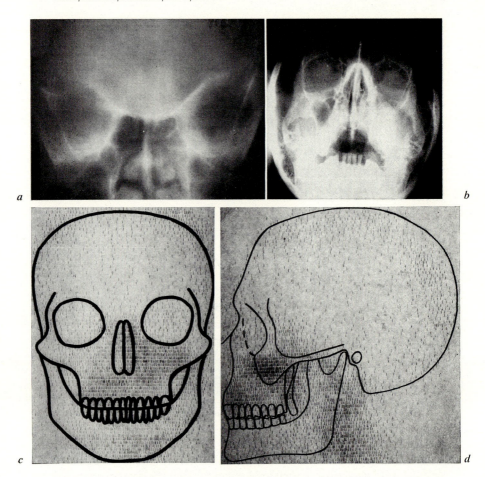

Fig.4. 65-year-old male. Carcinoma of the left maxillary sinus with intensive uptake over the whole left maxillary sinus. The superior and posterior part and also the hard palate are involved.

sclerosing sinusitis of maxillary sinus had a normal activity pattern despite extreme bone condensation. Surgery revealed granulation tissue mixed with calcium and bone, which was fixed to the posterior wall (this granulation tissue had to be chiselled from the posterior wall). On the other hand expansively growing osteomas of the maxillary sinus [7] may have as increased an abnormal uptake as an osteogeneous sarcoma.

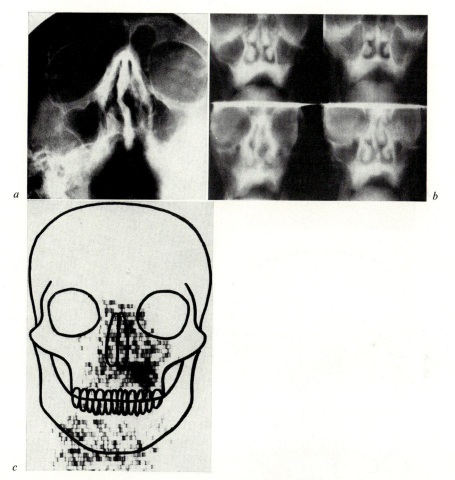

Fig. 5. 67-year-old male. Early diagnosis of a carcinoma of the left maxillary sinus and of the hard palate. There is a focally increased uptake over the lower third of the left maxillary sinus. The tomogram revealed a soft tissue density in the recessus alveolaris on both sides and a thinning of the left part of the hard palate. Biopsy showed a carcinoma.

Osteolysis, Osteoporosis

Lesions with Increased Uptake

There is intensive focally increased radionuclide uptake in projection on facial bones and the floor of the anterior cranial fossa.

(a) In acute osteomyelitis of the frontal sinus, maxilla and mandibula[9]. Especially in hematogeneous osteomyelitis [9] (fig. 10) the bone image was

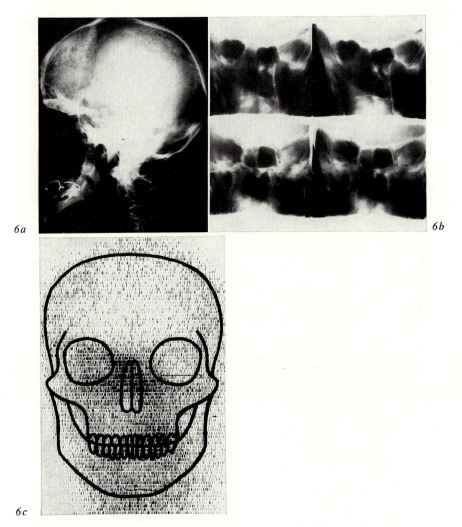

Fig.6. 69-year-old female. Recurrence in a patient with a carcinoma of the left maxillary sinus which was operated and irradiated in 1969. In 1975 surgery of the recurrence with total removal of the maxilla. In 1976 the parotis was removed and the floor of the mouth was resected. The intensive tracer accumulation over the middle skull base correponds to the new recurrence in the area of the sphenoid sinus.

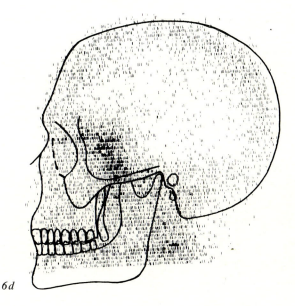

6d

very often found positive before any bone changes were evident in the tomograms. This aids in early diagnoses.

(b) In bone destructions of malignant tumors of maxillary sinus, orbita, frontal sinus, os maxillaris, os zygomaticum, hard palate and mandibula. The nuclide accumulation is independent of histology as carcinoma, sarcoma, malignant lymphoepithelioma, basalioma and cylindroma.

Destruction of Antral Walls

Destruction of maxillary antral walls demonstrates in all 11 cases a markedly increased uptake, either localized (fig. 5, 6) or generalized (fig. 4) according to the extent of the bone lesion. Well-defined focus of increased radioactivity of smaller lesions in the floor of the orbita, of the lateral, medial, anterior and posterior antral walls (fig. 5) could demonstrate the exact site. The localization of the lesion can be very accurate for surgical biopsy to diagnose early or as early as possible malignant tumors or the early recurrence of an already treated tumor, when there is radiographically only a homogeneous density of maxillary sinus and bone destruction is only questionable or totally absent (fig. 5). Destructions limited to the maxillary sinus have on lateral scan an increased uptake over the well-defined area of the sinus. Twelve patients had an expansion to the posterior ethmoid cells and sphenoid sinus and demonstrated an additional nuclide accumulation in projection to the floor of the

Table I. Comparison of bone imaging and tomography in 40 malignant tumors within the facial bones and of the skull base

	Radiogram and scans positive	More information on radiograms	on scans
Localization			
Maxillary sinus	10	1	1
Maxillary sinus + ethmoid bone	3	1	2
Maxillary sinus + sphenoid sinus	9	0	2
Ethmoid bone + sphenoid sinus	2	1	0
Frontal bone	1	1	0
Cavum nasi	2	0	0
Orbita	1	0	0
Ethmoid bone	1	1	0
Temporal bone	1	0	0
	30	5	5
Histology			
Carcinoma	20	2	3
Sarcoma	6	3	2
Plasmocytoma	1	0	0
Hemangiopericytoma	1	0	0
Lymphoepithelioma	2	0	0
	30	5	5

middle cerebral fossa. The radioactivity may be more intensive than that of the primary tumor. There was the tendency to invade the ethmoid and sphenoid sinuses (fig. 8). An additional increased uptake was seen on anterior scans centrally between both orbitae, when the maxillary sinus carcinoma expanded to the ethmoid cells and sphenoid sinus. Because these structures are projected over each other, both could be evaluated separately only on lateral view (fig. 8).

Tumor invasions to the cavum nasi, the opposite sinus and orbita demonstrate often a band-like or a round focal increased activity pattern. While on the radiogram there is only a homogeneous softtissue density, the scan allows to find out the areas with the highest tumor activity (fig. 8). The altered osteogenesis is often more extended on the scan than radiographically supposed. So tomography illustrates osteolysis at the caudal and medial wall of the orbita, while the scan may bring out an additional osteolysis at the lateral and superior wall. The exact involvement gained by scans is of great value for planning surgery or follow-up after treatment.

Table II. Comparison of bone scan and tomography in 24 benign tumors within the facial bones and of the skull base

	Radiogram and scan positive	More information on radiogram
Localization		
Maxillary sinus	1	2
Maxillary sinus + ethmoid bone	1	2
Maxillary sinus + sphenoid sinus	5	2
Ethmoid bone + sphenoid sinus	2	0
Frontal bone	2	3
Orbita	3	0
Occipital bone	0	1
	14	10
Histology		
Osteoma	6	4
Polyposis	1	1
Chondroma	1	0
Angiofibroma	0	1
Cylindroma	3	2
Osteogeneous fibroma	1	1
Fibroma	1	0
Basalioma	1	1
	14	10

Primary Malignant Tumor of Cavum nasi and of Ethmoid Sinus

In contrast to the laterally situated destructions of the maxillary sinus, destructions within the cavum nasi and ethmoid cells are difficult to diagnose on the scans, because the maximum activity is normally in the center and in this case the comparison with the uninvolved opposite side is impossible.

Two patients with carcinoma of the cavum nasi showed an osteolysis markedly more extensive on one side. Comparing the uninvolved side the scan showed a focal, well-defined area of increased radioactivity at the destruction. In all cases the activity was markedly increased at the facial bones on the lateral scan. Out of two primary malignant tumors of the ethmoid cells one carcinoma did not reveal an increased uptake, while one sarcoma had a 2-cm diameter intensive tracer accumulation in the center, seen on a.-p. and lateral scan. A huge plasmocytoma involving the cavum nasi and ethmoid cells with soft tissue swelling demonstrated only a slightly increased uptake over the cavum nasi without a preponderance of a circumscript area.

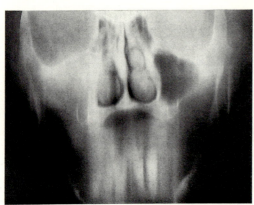
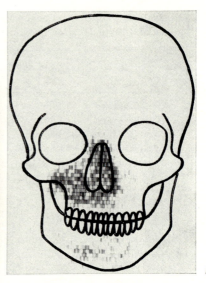

a   *b*

Fig. 7. 63-year-old female. Intensive soft tissue fixation of ⁹⁹ᵐTc-phosphate compounds within the newly formed granulation tissue and polypoid tissue in the right sinus maxillaris and in the right cavum nasi as a result of a foreign body irritation by a not resorbable cortisol-sulfonamide package in a chronic sinusitis maxillaris

Benign lesions

A very intensive tracer uptake is found in osteochondroma with osteolysis and expansive growth [17]. It may balloon out and destroy the walls of the maxillary sinus. We saw increased tracer accumulation in a chondroma of the orbita associated with osteolysis, in a polyposis nasi and in a fibroma of the maxillary sinus, of the frontal sinus and of the ethmoid cells. The latter did not show an erosion in tomography.

We also got a very marked increase in uptake over the maxillary sinus and cavum nasi in two patients with rapidly growing granulation tissue as a foreign body reaction according to a not absorbable antibiotic package put in 3 weeks earlier because of chronic sinusitis maxillaris (fig. 7). In contrast to most malignant bone destructions there was an accumulation over the maxillary sinus not more marked than that over the cavum nasi. At surgery the bone was intact. The abnormally increased radionuclide deposition of ⁹⁹ᵐTc-tin-phosphate compound was also exclusively in soft tissue. The granulation tissue contains a lot of newly formed collagen, to which the ⁹⁹ᵐTc compound is adsorbed [3, 16] and is found to a fair extent in the osteoid and in the pannus. Extra-osseous increased accumulation of ⁹⁹ᵐTc compound is

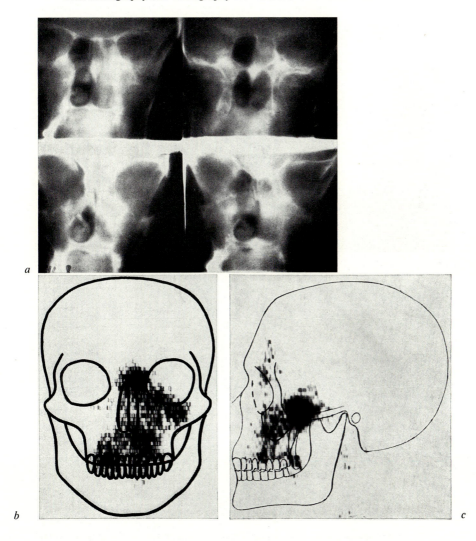

Fig.8. 70-year-old female. A primary carcinoma of the left sinus maxillaris invades the middle of the skull base, the frontal bone and the right maxillary sinus. Some areas with focally increased bone metabolism with a tracer maximum over the middle skull base on the lateral scan.

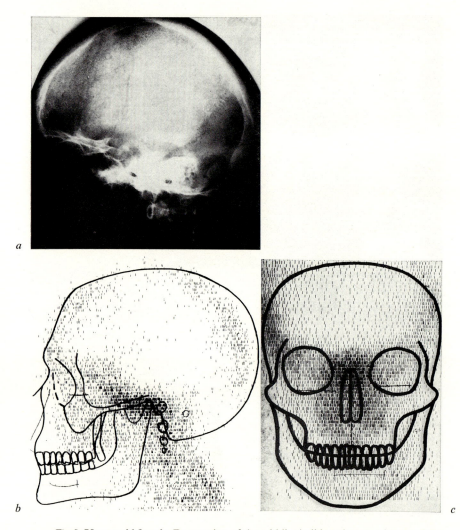

Fig. 9. 75-year-old female. Destruction of the middle skull base by a carcinoma of the epipharynx. Very intensive accumulation over the middle skull base with a maximum over the sphenoid bone seen in the center without lateralization on the a.p. scan.

also demonstrated in inflammatory serous fluids, in abscesses, in amyloid tissue, in brain and myocardial infarctions, in intramuscular Fe-dextran compounds, in irradiated tissue, in some soft tissue tumors, in lung tumors in lymphomas and in adenocarcinoma of the liver.

3 h after a preoperative injection of ^{99m}Tc in an intraoperative resected

tissue of a reticulumcell sarcoma of the cavum nasi, we found an increased uptake in the adjacent inflammatory tumor-free tissue in a 2:1 ratio and in the resected bone in a 7:1 ratio to the uninvolved, intact tissue. The more proliferating margin of an epidermoid carcinoma had an increased uptake in a 3:1 ratio to the center of the tumor.

Lesions with Absent or Less Nuclide Uptake

Very slowly growing, benign soft tissue tumors did not show an increased accumulation when they expanded but did not infiltrate the walls, as a 5 cm in diameter, big, juvenile angiofibroma of a 17-year-old boy, which had encased the maxillary sinus to one third from dorsolateral. Mucoceles of the maxillary sinus demonstrated an absent or only slightly increased accretion. Sometimes a fair lateralization of an increased uptake on the involved area was seen, but never as marked as in destructions of the sinus wall by malignant tumors. The scans of 25 acute or subacute maxillary, ethmoid or sphenoid sinusitises revealed either normal or slightly increased uptake, which is never as intensive as in malignant destructions (fig. 4, 8), osteoplastic tumors (fig. 2), systemic diseases with increased bone metabolism (fig. 3) or acute osteomyelitis (fig. 10). But sometimes malignant lesions also have only a slightly increased nuclide uptake. In this case the history, the clinical examination and finally the biopsy may contribute to the diagnosis.

The Floor of the Middle Cerebral Fossa

Tumors invading the middle cerebral fossa from facial bones and from the anterior part of the skull base demonstrated, besides the ventrally increased uptake, an additional very marked tracer accumulation over the area of the sphenoid sinus on lateral scans (fig. 3). The bone destructions of the sinus and greater wing of the os sphenoidale had an increased uptake in the center and lateral edge respectively depending on the site on anterior scans. An increased uptake over the middle cerebral fossa without further accumulation is seen when a tumor of the epipharynx or from the parotic area invades the floor of the middle cerebral fossa. This scan may therefore resemble that of a primary tumor or of an osteolytic metastasis in that area [6, 11]. Despite cranial nerve paresis the radiograms may be normal. The scan, however, may show localized focally increased uptake. Osteoplastic and ossifying tumors, such as osteoma, osteogeneous sarcoma and ossifying fibroma have a very dense accumulation.

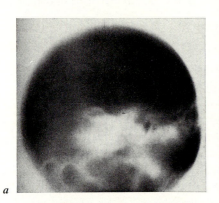
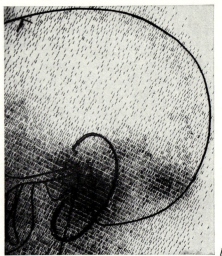

a *b*

Fig. 10. 62-year-old male. Otitis externa necroticans with facial nerve paresis. There was a strong nuclide accumulation over the left ear on the scan. The tomogram did not show any pathological changes.

Posterior Cerebral Fossa

In contrast to the mostly sagittal and parasagittal lesions in the middle cerebral fossa, lesions of the posterior fossa have the increased uptake laterally for anatomical reasons. A relatively slight difference in tracer accumulation of both sides is discernible on a.-p. scans, but it is difficult to separate the lesion on a lateral scan, because the maximum of activity is in projection over the ear. A laterally localized increased uptake was seen in a destruction by a malignant tumor of the temporal bone, which was also demonstrated on tomograms [7, 8] and in some tomographically hardly demonstrable arrosions of the petrous apex, e. g. by a tumor of the epipharynx and in a tomographically negative destruction by a osteomyelitis of the external ear in a 62-year-old patient with diabetes and facial paresis (fig. 10). On the other hand only a tomogram revealed a 1 cm in diameter metastatic osteolysis in the canalis nervi hypoglossi, where the scan and the plain radiograms were normal. These examples support the contributory value of both the tomography and the nuclear medicine diagnosis bone lesions. The scan reveals especially the bone metabolism and detects areas with increased uptake, i. e. with increased osteogenesis. The value of bone imaging of the facial bones and of the floor of the skull base in comparison with tomography is summarized.

Summary

(1) Bone scans permit sometimes the early diagnosis of osteomyelitis, bone metastases and bone destructions by tumors before changes are visited on radiograms. (2) Scans with localized focal increased activity extend the radiographic diagnosis when bone destructions are questionable on tomography. (3) Bone imaging improves the radiographic diagnosis of tumor recurrence after surgery, radiation therapy and medical treatment through isotope follow-up, when tomography shows homogeneous soft tissue density or unchanged anatomical morphology. (4) The scan demonstrates the most suitable site for bone biopsy through areas of abnormal nuclide accumulation as a sign of locally increased bone metabolism, when tomography shows a homogeneous density. (5) Scanning determines the exact tumor extension and aids in planning surgery and radiation therapy, because the bone metabolism may be more extensive on scintigraphs than the bone changes on radiograms. (6) The scan helps to detect local different bone metabolism activity with different increased accumulation in comparison to homogeneous changes on tomograms. (7) The scan may show a local invasion to adjacent bones or to the base of the skull. (8) Scintigraphic follow-up studies give information on the success of treatment after surgery, irradiation and medical treatment. Healed bone diseases show a progressive tendency to a normal activity pattern, but recurrences show a more increased uptake. (9) Bone scanning aids in differential diagnosis of malignant lesions and inflammation of paranasal sinuses. A very increased uptake exludes practically a sinusitis, but a slightly increased activity pattern is unequivocal.

References

1   Boszo, G. und Fornet, B.: Vergleichende Röntgen- und Knochenszintigraphie-Untersuchungen der Nebenhöhlenerkrankungen. Kongressband Dt. Öster. Röntgenges. Wien 1973, p. 263 (Thieme, Stuttgart 1974).

2   Büll, U. und Frey, K.W.: Nuklearmedizinische Methoden in der Diagnostik von Knochenerkrankungen. Internist *16:* 353–364 (1975).

3   Büll, U.; Lieven, B. v. und Leisner, B.: Zur Frage der Weichteilkonzentration von ^{99m}Tc-Zinn-Phosphat-Komplexen. Nukl-Med. *14:* 91–105 (1975).

4   Frey, K.W.; Sonntag, A.; Scheybani, M.S.; Krauss, O. und Fuchs, P.: Knochenszintigraphie mit Strontium 85. Fortschr. Röntgenstr. *106:* 206–215 (1967).

5   Frey, K.W.: Profilmessung und Szintigraphie des Skeletts; in Glauner Angiologie und Szintigraphie bei Knochen- und Gelenkserkrankungen (Thieme, Stuttgart 1971).

6   FREY, K.W.: Tomographie des Gesichtsschädels und des Kiefergelenkes. Kontrast-
     mitteldarstellung und Isotope. Bayer. Zahnärztebl. *1970:* 137–147.

7   FREY, K.W.; BÜLL, U.; HUEBER, M.; HEENEMANN, H. und MÜNZEL, M.: Szintigraphie
     mit ^{99m}Tc-Pyrophosphat, ^{99m}Tc-Polyphosphat, ^{87m}Sr und Profilmessungen mit ^{85}Sr
     im Vergleich mit der Röntgen-Tomographie bei Erkrankungen des Gesichtsschädels
     und der Schädelbasis. Kongressband 'Nuklearmedizin'. 11.Tag.Ges.Nuklearmed.,
     Athen 1973, pp.453–458 (Schattauer, Stuttgart 1974).

8   FREY, K.W.; HUEBER, M.; MÜNZEL, M. und ROHLOFF, R.: Szintigraphie bei Tumoren
     und entzündlichen Prozessen der Schädelbasis. Röntgen-Ber. *5:* 171–192 (1976).

9   HEENENMANN, R.: Profilmessung und Szintigraphie des Schädels mit Radiostrontium;
     Inaug. Diss. München (1971).

10   HÖR, G.; FREY, K.W. und PABST, H.W.: Szintigraphie von Tumoren im Kopf-Hals-
     Bereich. Zahnärztebl. *25:* 204–209 (1971).

11   LANGHAMMER, H. and FREY, K.W.: Tumor scintigraphy with radiogallium and radio-
     strontium. J. dentomaxillofac. Radiol. *1:* 30 (1972).

12   MÜNZEL, M.; FREY, K.W. und BÜLL, U.: Szintigraphische Untersuchungen des Ge-
     sichtsschädels. Arch.Ohr.-Nas.-KehlkHeilk. *205:* 345–348 (1973).

13   MÜNZEL, M.; FREY, K.W. und BÜLL, U.: Die diagnostische Wertigkeit der Knochen-
     szintigraphie des Gesichtsschädels. Öst. Ärztetag. *30:* 1305 (1975).

14   REISNER, K. und GOSEPATH, J.: Schädeltomographie (Thieme, Stuttgart 1973).

15   ROSENTHALL, L. and KAYE, M.: Technetium-99m-pyrophosphate kinetics and imaging
     in metabolic bone disease. J. nucl. Med. *16:* 33 (1975).

16   SUBRAMANIAN, G.; McAFEE, J.G.; BELL, E.G.; BLAIR, R.J.; O'MARA, R.E., and
     RASTON, P.H.: ^{99m}Tc-labeled polyphosphate as a skeletal imaging agent. Radiology
     102: 701 (1972).

17   WICKENHAUSER, J. v.; STRASSL, H. und HOLLMANN, K.: Das benigne Osteoblastom.
     Fortschr. Röntgenstr. *119:* 618–623 (1973).

Prof. Dr. K.W. FREY, Zentrale Röntgenabteilung, Universitäts-Poliklinik, Pettenkofer-
strasse 8a, *D-8000 München 2* (FRG)